History of Yoga

It All Started on a Stone

Ramis Kachar

document is for educational and entertainment purposes only. All effort has been executed to present accurate, up to date, reliable, complete information. No warranties of any kind are declared or implied. Readers acknowledge that the author is not engaging in the rendering of legal, financial, medical or professional advice. The content within this book has been derived from various sources. Please consult a licensed professional before attempting any techniques outlined in this book.

By reading this document, the reader agrees that under no circumstances is the author responsible for any losses, direct or indirect, that are incurred as a result of the use of information contained within this document, including, but not limited to, errors, omissions, or inaccuracies.

Authors Note

The purpose of this book is to share information that I have learnt and practiced over many years on my Yoga journey. As a Yoga Historian, a teacher and a student.

After reading many ancient texts, books and journals I wanted to share the information but in a clear and simple manor so as to be easy and enjoyable to read and understand, for those who are and who are not avid followers of Yoga.

Yoga can have a place for all of us in our lives and although that may sound like a brash statement, I am confident this will be clear after reading this book.

From being a person who judged Yoga with a narrow view when first introduced to finding the whole history and purpose to be truly fascinating, I hope you do too.

Table of Content

Introduction

Whether you've walked through a gym or community center, or whether you've learned about it from your friends, you're probably familiar with the popularity of yoga. In the U.S., yoga has quite a following, and at this point, it's supported as an exercise and a way to achieve an overall sense of well-being. Depending on who you ask, you will get so many different definitions of yoga. It could be something simple as, "That class of women who do the stretchy things," or intense like, "The spiritual center of my soul." Really. Every person gets something out of yoga and so their definitions will reflect that.

With a definition like that, it's hard to know what yoga is exactly. And with that question comes another one, why is yoga so popular? I mean, you can't walk down a city block without coming across either a person headed toward a yoga class, or a yoga studio, or a gym that has a yoga class, etc. So why is it popular and where did it come from? How has yoga dominated the scene for so long?

This book will help you with these questions. While there are many books out there on the topic, they're not easy to read. There are some great books out there, but many of them are written from a research perspective, each of them filled with difficult philosophy lessons, difficult language, and a lot of extra information that may not be easily read. They're often written with researchers or those already steeped on yoga philosophy in mind. While these books are all worthy and very interesting reads, we understand the need to have yoga explained in a more manageable way. This is that book. The goal of this book is to show you the history of yoga, with clear, easy to follow explanations. We'll go over the origins of yoga, and talk about some of the key ancient texts associated. All of this is set up in an easy-to-understand manner for modern audiences. We'll go over all of your burning yoga questions and talk about yoga's development over the last 7000 years. Yes, it is that ancient. But its history will surprise you and hopefully relieve some of your unanswered questions.

Now that we've covered what this book is about, let me explain a little about why I wrote it. I'm just like a lot of other people out there. I started practicing yoga because I learned from a friend that it would help me get stronger and more flexible. For me, yoga was entirely about being pain free and being able to move without creaks in my body. When I first started yoga, it was because I was concerned over my range of motion, my stiffness, and my aches and pains. I definitely wasn't expecting age to affect me like this, especially when I still considered myself young at 30! So yoga was my solution.

When I first walked through the door to the yoga class, I was a little worried about how I would fair. After all, I wasn't like those fit, athletic people in the videos or ads for yoga. But my worry quickly drifted away. The class opened a door for me. It created a community of supportive people, new friends, and also a love of yoga itself. As I got better at the poses, I started learning more about the rituals and philosophy behind yoga. It was a fascinating world for me.

From that point on, I wanted to learn as much as I could about yoga and I decided to learn from the "home country." So I traveled to India and Nepal to learn what I could. I researched a lot of history, and also started teaching others about what I learned. However, one thing that surprised me was just the sheer amount of speculation about yoga history.

You see, most of the history associated with yoga was shared through oral tradition. This means there weren't any books until much later. So what we know about ancient yoga now is a mix of research based on saved texts, translations, remnants of oral tradition, and best guesses. All of this was interesting to me, and so I thought it might be interesting to others as well. That's where this book comes into play.

Now, you dear reader, may be like me. You may be practicing yoga right now, or you may want to practice it in the future. Or perhaps you may be someone who has no intention of ever practicing. Either which way, your curious mind has brought you here. I honestly believe that knowing the history behind yoga can help with understanding our own practices more. Even if you don't practice, knowing the background of yoga can help with knowing the human experience and the 'self' more. It can change our perception of our everyday actions and events and if we apply what we've learned about yoga, we can experience immense emotional, physical, mental, and spiritual growth.

Throughout my journey, I've learned that yoga is more than just physical postures and that there is a rich culture of spiritual and mental wellbeing behind it. This knowledge has enriched my own practice and I hope that it can enrich yours too. Knowing the history gave me an opportunity to fine tune my physical practice, but also helped me with my mindset. I started to understand the purpose of meditation and the breaths during yoga practice. I also started to have more respect for the importance of mental wellbeing and how yoga can help with it.

As yoga keeps increasing in popularity, I feel that it's important for all of us to go back and look at the roots of it. It's important not to forget it's origins and why it was developed. But more than this, knowing the origins can have practical applications today.

This book will help you in your search for knowledge. I'll draw from sources like ancient texts, researchers, and historians to help explain the history of yoga. We'll go into the development of yoga during each era in the Indian subcontinent and we'll touch on every aspect that aided the development of yoga. By the end of the book, you'll have a new perspective on yoga. I promise that you'll learn at least one new thing from this book, and hopefully be able to apply some of what's learned to your current life. After all, learning new things is how we grow as a people, and I honestly believe the history of yoga and the ancient aspects of it will help you do that.

The information here is written in an easy to understand way, but it would also be a good idea to read it again a few times, just so that it's fully understood. Take the time to process what is learned and consider whether its applicable to your modern lifestyle.

Chapter 1

What's all the Fuss About

I bet if you walked into your workplace right now, and asked how many people practice yoga, about one-third of your workplace would raise their hands. Yoga is incredibly popular today and there are many people who practice it. From your grandmother to your dog walker, there are at least two people in your life who practice yoga. If you're reading this book, it's likely that you practice yoga, or you're interested in practicing it. You're not alone. There are roughly 36 million people in the U.S. who practice yoga, and that's a statistic from three years ago (Wei, 2016). Could you imagine how many people practice now? The answer is a lot. I know that's not scientific, but it's a lot. You can't even drive around a city block without seeing a yoga studio.

Yoga is a practice that is enjoyed across the lifespan. Children, teens, adults, and seniors can all enjoy the benefits of yoga and there are classes and practices dedicated to each age group. While we generally see young, thin women in yoga ads, yoga is enjoyed by everyone. In fact, middle-aged adults and seniors practice yoga far more than youths. If you are healthy and fit, or not, you can still benefit from yoga practice.

Despite all the popularity and the endorsements from celebrities about the wonder of yoga, it's hard to know exactly what yoga is exactly. After all, is yoga just stretching? How is it different from other stretches? What makes it so popular? These are questions that we'll address in this chapter.

What is Yoga?

Yoga is a detailed, beautifully historic practice. We'll get into how it developed during later chapters, but today, yoga is most easily recognized as a meditative exercise. When I say 'meditative exercise,' I use the phrase to show both aspects of yoga. Yoga can be used for mindfulness and meditation, but it's also used for physical exercise. So there are often two parts to yoga, the physical and the spiritual. Let's look at both parts.

Physical exercise

Most of us are aware of yoga as an exercise. When you go to a mainstream yoga class, this is what you typically get. Yoga for exercise is all about moving your muscles and holding stretches to increase your flexibility. It doesn't really matter what type of yoga you do, there is always this element of stretching and some holding, even if it's only for a breath. Whether your practice is slow or fast, you'll have poses that align your body in certain ways to give you relief, or to cause you to stretch tight muscle groups. By the end of many yoga sessions, you feel loose, light, and often relaxed. If you're doing an active practice, you may even feel worn out.

Yoga works with all muscle groups. For beginners, most of your poses are going to focus on the legs, arms, hips, and some chest poses. Once you move to more advanced poses, you start to work on all parts of your body, stretching your back, shoulders, abdominals, and more. You can even do yoga that focuses on your hands, feet, neck, and head. So yoga can activate as many muscles as other kinds of physical exercise.

There is a strength component to yoga, though it's more subtle than say lifting weights. This is because it uses your own body weight to increase your strength. People can often add extra parts to yoga for increased strength development, but for the most part, your body weight in specific poses is all there is. The poses help your body to build more strength in each muscle group. They also help to increase your flexibility by reducing muscle stiffness. Of course, just like many other exercises, depending on the type of yoga you do, you may walk away from the session and be sore the next day.

While most of us see yoga as a strength building or flexibility building exercise, it's also a cardio-vascular exercise. Cardio exercises, often called aerobics, help improve your heart health and circulatory health. Running, cycling, and swimming are all exercises that get your heart racing and in turn help to improve your cardiovascular health. Yoga can also do the same. While there are many slow yoga practices, there are also some very intense ones. There are yoga practices that move very quickly, moving from pose to pose and putting you in strenuous positions. These often cause your heart to race and for you to start sweating as you strain in each position. This cardiovascular benefit is even better if the practice is done for a long duration (think an hour long class instead of a 15 minute one). So yoga can also be considered a cardiovascular exercise if it's done with that goal in mind.

The breath also plays a key role in the physical aspects of yoga. You'll often find when you do exercise that you breath as you like. More often than not, you're breathing shallowly and rapidly if you're doing cardio and sometimes you might even hold your breath when you do other kinds of exercise. In yoga, there is emphasis on the breath, your aim could be to breathe slowly, or sometimes quickly, but always deeply. This helps you to maintain focus as you go through your poses, but also helps connect each movement to a breath. This means that your timing is naturally orientated. It also helps you to truly focus on the 'hows' of your practice. You start to pay more attention to the movement of your shoulders or hips, how your back is positioned, or the angle of your joints. All of this can lead to better, safer, pose positions, but also help strengthen the rest of your body.

So yoga is a physical exercise that goes beyond just stretching. It offers strength and flexibility training and cardiovascular training. These things are more than just average stretching which most newcomers expect. Incorporating the right breathing also brings you better stability and balance, which are important to most exercises.

Mental and spiritual exercise

Beyond the physical aspects of yoga are the mental and spiritual aspects. Mentally, yoga practice can put you in a 'zone'. You know the zone I'm talking about. It's the zone of perfect focus. Maybe you've experienced the 'zone' at work, when you're working on a perfect project and you are utterly focused on your task. This focus helps you to achieve more. In different circumstances, it can help you engage with others and to quiet the anxiety in your mind. This focus is incredibly beneficial. During a yoga practice, you might find yourself slipping into that perfect 'zone', where your mind is quiet and you are fully focused on your body's movement. A lot of people call it a sense of peace when they practice, whether it's a slow yoga practice or a quick one.

Yoga also provides another aspect to that focus. It often provides awareness. Awareness is not just a general awareness of the events in the current day. In combination with focus, awareness means that you are aware of your present moment, what is happening around you and inside of you. This presents a type of clarity. Instead of thinking about what you are going to do later on in the day, or stressing about what you did the day before, you are placed in this present moment. A consistent yoga practice can often lead to this moment. So yoga can increase your focus and awareness inside practice, but these are lessons you can also carry with you.

A key part of achieving awareness and focus during yoga practice is your breathing. Yes, just like when we discussed how the breath affects you physically, it also affects you mentally. By actively choosing to focus on your breathing, you move the function from one that's automatic to one that is consciously thought about. This is very similar to mindfulness, where you focus on the breathing and exclude some of the other thoughts in your mind. Yoga can put you into a mindful state while you are practicing. By focusing on the breath and poses, you move your mind away from emotional stress and focus it instead on the present moment and actions. This results in that feeling of being 'lifted' that many people feel after doing a yoga session. That being said, you don't want to focus on the breath so much that you end up feeling drained at the end of the session. Balance is key.

The mindfulness and meditative aspects of yoga are closely related to spirituality. Spirituality is different from religion, though they do tend to be mistaken for one another. Spirituality is about your connection to the fundamental life questions. Mindfulness and meditation can be a part of spirituality. They can also be a part of religion if you practice a religion where mindfulness and meditation are encouraged. Religions, unlike general spirituality, is about your connection to a fundamental power and usually includes religious texts and rituals. If you are religious, it generally (though not always) affects your spirituality. But if you're spiritual, that doesn't necessarily mean you're religious.

I don't really want to get into the philosophical aspects of religion and spirituality. Suffice it to say that activities that help clear the mind, like yoga, are often considered to be a part of spirituality since they take you beyond yourself and instead help you focus on the moment now. That being said, yoga is only spiritual if that's how you want it to be. For many people, they only want the physical aspects of yoga, and others practice purely for the spiritual or religious aspects. If you're more interested in the connection between yoga and spirituality or religion, then the final chapter of this book will explore that topic more in depth.

Whatever your reasoning for practicing yoga, you can call it an exercise that is both physical and spiritual, which moves it a bit beyond your typical exercise experience.

What Happens in a Yoga Class?

Start your yoga class journey by first finding a class with a trained yoga instructor. This should be someone who has a lot of experience in both yoga and understanding the body. If you have a yoga instructor who is properly trained, they'll know how to provide variations for your skill levels, position your body correctly to avoid injury, and they won't ask you to do poses that put you at risk for injury. If your yoga instructor seems like they're not offering these things, then find another place to go.

In your yoga class, your mat will be rolled out and you will be facing the instructor. Before the class starts, talk to your instructor about any injuries you have, so they can offer you some variations for different poses.

Once the class starts, you're going to be involved in different poses. Your instructor might call them out in their English form, but they may also use the Sanskrit form. Here are a few that you'll experience in your typical yoga class, with the titles listed with both the English names and the Sanskrit ones. While these are fairly common poses, whether you see them in class or not depends on whether the class is for beginning or advanced students, with some of these poses in advanced classes only. Here you go:

- **Downward dog (Adho Mukha Svan-asana):** Downward dog is one of the most familiar yoga pose. In downward dog, you make an inverted 'v' with your head, torso, and arms down one side of the 'v' and your legs on the other. It's used frequently as a part of various sequences. It's generally considered a beginner pose, and has many variations that people can work with. It exercises and strengthens the legs and arms.

This is a foundational yoga pose, which means that it's one that you should know and position well since it often leads into other poses in a sequence.

- **Upward facing dog (Urdhva Mukha Svanasana):** Upward dog is a pose where you start on your front and then raise your body off the floor with only your hand and the tops of your feet touching the mat. It seems easy, but can also cause some back pain if done incorrectly, so it's considered an intermediate or advanced pose. It exercises and strengthens the arms. If you are a beginner, don't go into upward dog until you've already strengthened your back. Instead, try the cobra pose (below).

- **Mountain pose (Tadasana):** Mountain pose is often the first pose in a sequence. It seems like it just requires you to stand up, but it's more than that. For mountain pose, you want to bring awareness to your position. Make sure you spine is long and straight and that you feel the mat with each 'corner' of your feet. Mountain pose is considered a beginner pose and is often restorative. Being restorative, it means it doesn't strengthen a particular muscle group, but it does help if you need a break from one of the harder poses. It's a great pose to revert to if you want to catch your breath. Mountain pose is a foundational pose, meaning that you should practice and have it set since it's often the pose used in the beginning or middle of a harder sequence.

- **Warrior I, II, and III (Virabhadrasana I, II, III):** Warriors I, II, and III are all poses that require you to be in a type of lunge or balanced position on one foot. They get progressively harder as you transition from one to the other. You often won't use all three in a sequence, but maybe one or two, depending on the class you're in. Warrior I and II are considered beginner poses and Warrior III is considered more intermediate or advanced. All the poses will strengthen your legs, core, and hips. While they seem easy if you see a photo, it's a good idea to practice them first with a trained yoga teacher so you can get the positioning just right. If your hips are out of alignment, then it can cause you pain later on.

- **Cat-Cow pose (Marjaryasana-Bitil-asana):** Cat-cow pose is very popular and is often used as a warmup in gentle yoga or children's yoga. For the pose, you start in a hands and knees position and then arch your back like a cat, followed by bowing your back, like a cow. It's a great exercise to warm up your back, especially your lower back. Cat-cow pose is considered a beginners pose and exercises your core, back, and chest muscles. To shift from cat to cow, make sure that you follow your breaths.

- **Chair pose (Utkatasana):** The best way to describe chair pose is that you are sitting on an imaginary chair with your hands holding an imaginary ball above your head. Needless to say, chair pose is considered an intermediate pose since it requires some considerable core strength. It's a pose that can be learned, and if you're use to doing squats, then chair pose will be a breeze. Chair pose strengthens the legs, spine, and core muscles.

- **Plank:** If you are familiar with body-weight exercises, then plank will also be familiar. It is used in yoga as a core strengthening pose. Since it's held for a couple of breaths, or quickly used before progressing into another pose, it's considered an intermediate pose. To hold it, you'll need a lot of core strength and arm strength. Plank is a foundational pose that brings you into other poses. It's often used during the sun salutation sequence. If you're new to plank, it's a good idea to have a yoga trainer set you up, since you want to avoid locking your joints and make sure that your lower back is strong.

- **Cobra pose (Bhujangasana):** Cobra pose is like a baby upward dog. It doesn't require you to lift your whole body off the floor like upward dog does, so it's a good starter pose. In this pose, you are facing downwards with your lower body pressed into the mat and your torso is lifted up, with you resting on your hands. Cobra pose is considered to be a beginner pose, and as I mentioned before, it's a good practice pose to get you into upward dog. Cobra pose helps you strength-en the spine and chest. If you have a weaker back, you'll want to take care during the pose, since it requires a bend in your lower back.

- **Forward fold (Uttanasana):** Forward fold is a bend at the hips from a standing position with the chest pressed firmly against the thighs. It stretches the backs of your legs and your hips. Forward fold is considered to be a beginner pose, and is also a foundational one, since it leads to many other poses. If you ever feel worn out while doing standing poses (like the Warrior poses), then you can always rest in forward fold, as it keeps your body engaged and upright, but is also a fairly restful pose.

- **Knees, Chest, Chin (Ashtanga Namaskara):** This pose is a lying down pose, with the chin, chest, and knees touching the mat, and you braced on your hands. It's a good pose to practice before getting into four-limbed staff (another pose). Because it requires you to have significant bends in your neck and back, it's a good idea to have a yoga instructor position you first so you know how it's supposed to be performed before using it. Despite all of this, it's considered a beginner pose since it isn't hard to maintain. It stretches your back and arms.

- **Four-limbed staff (Chaturanga Dandasana):** This pose is like a plank, but lower to the ground, with you resting on your hands and toes. Unlike a plank, which has your arms under your shoulders and fully extended, four-limbed staff is a pose where your arms are on the side of your body. Your elbows are at a 90 degree angle with your upper arm parallel to the floor and your forearms perpendicular. It's an advanced pose...if you didn't already get that from the description. It requires a lot of arm strength to maintain, so a good idea is to use knees, chest, chin pose to practice first. Usually from this pose you move into downward or upward dog. It strengthens your arms, wrists, and core muscles.

- **Child's pose (Balasana):** Child's pose is considered to be a restful pose and is usually used at the end of a sequence or whenever you need a break in the sequence. It's a little hard to describe what it looks like, but generally if you were sitting on your knees and then bending forward until your forehead touches the floor, that's close to child's pose. Child's pose is considered to be a beginners pose, since it doesn't require a lot of preparation and can be easily adapted to all flexibility levels. It gently stretches the back and your hips. When you're in the pose, you tend to feel some relief as it's a pose that requires you to rest on your heels with your body nestled between your thighs.

- **Triangle pose (Trikonasana):** Triangle pose is called such because your legs make a triangle, with one leg extended forwards, and the other back. Your hips are the pivot point of the triangle and the mat makes the bottom edge. In the pose, your hands are vertical, perpendicular to the floor, with one hand resting on the floor and the other raised up into the air. Because triangle pose requires a significant amount of balance and flexibility, it's considered an intermediate-advanced pose. It often follows or is a part of a warrior pose sequence. Triangle pose strengthens the legs, hips, spine, chest, and shoulders (that's a lot!). Because it's a more advanced pose, if you're a beginner, it's a good idea to have a partner or your yoga instructor there to help position you properly and help you maintain your balance.

- **Lotus pose (Padmasana)**: Lotus pose is often the sitting pose that many yogis sit in. It's a meditative pose with both legs folded into the creases of the knees, with the feet resting on top of the thighs. Essentially, it requires a deep bend and a lot of flexibility. It's considered an advanced pose because of how much stretch it has. It can negatively affect your knees and hips if you haven't increased your flexibility before, so please don't do it unless you have a very experienced teacher working with you to go through the progressive positions.

- **Corpse pose (Savasana):** Though the name is kinda off putting, it's fairly accurate. Basically, lie down and pretend you're dead. Let every muscle relax from your toes all the way up to the top of your head. Have your arms and legs relaxed. It's a very restorative pose and gives you the opportunity to practice your deep breathing. Because it's a simple position to be in, it's considered a beginners pose. However, don't let the position fool you. Just because it is simple in the sense you just lie down, doesn't mean that it's easy. Your body has to be in a neutral position, with all of the muscles relaxed, including the ones you don't ever think about, like your tongue, throat, forehead, and eyebrows. Many yoga sessions end with corpse pose or child's pose.

Depending on your class, you may go through various sequences of poses, or you might just rest in a couple of poses. Your instructor will call them out and the group will follow. Your instructor will also give recommendations for breathing patterns. If you're confused, don't worry. Your instructor will likely help you by walking around and giving suggestions to improved your position, or alternative poses. You can also look at the other people around you to get an idea of what to do or what variations you can do. This said, if in doubt seek the advice of the instructor.

We'll explore the different kinds of yoga in a later chapter, but for now, here are two common yoga sequences. These are for mostly intermediate level or higher yoga practitioners.

1. Warrior Sequence: Mountain pose, Warrior I, Humble Warrior, Warrior II, Reverse Warrior, Warrior III,
2. Sun Salutation: Mountain pose, raised arm pose, forward bend, flat back, plank, ashtanga namaskara, cobra pose, downward facing dog, forward bend, flat back, then end with mountain pose.

At the end of the class, your teacher will probably ask everyone to go into corpse pose, and then end the class with a 'Namaste,' which means "I bow to the Divine in you." And thus ends your yoga class!

Benefits of Yoga

Yoga has often been touted as a cure-all for each type of disease out there. This isn't exactly true, but instead, yoga may provide a very effective placebo effect. This means that when we're doing yoga, we're more likely to believe that we are healthier. This in turn helps us to actually be healthier. It's a surprisingly wonderful trick of our brains. Outside of this placebo effect, there are some benefits of yoga that have been researched. Here are some of the key benefits of yoga, many of which were first taught when yoga first came into existence.

Improved well-being

In general, yoga can improve your well-being. It's a great way to reduce the risk of many diseases, because yoga is exercise, and exercise is preventative in nature. To start with, yoga helps with your heart health. It's been shown that people who practice yoga often have reduced blood pressure. This leads to a healthier heart. Even simple relaxation poses like corpse poses can help you reduce your blood pressure (as cited in McCall, 2017). Yoga can also lead to a reduction in cholesterol and blood sugar levels. Like most exercises, yoga is incredibly beneficial for your heart health, and this in turn is connected to your overall well-being.

Another positive aspect of yoga is how it may affect your weight management. When you are practicing yoga, you tend to gain the benefits of mindfulness which can follow you home once the session is over. This mindfulness can help you be mindful about other areas in your life, like how you eat. Whe_ applying mindfulness to your relationship to food, it's likely that you'll have better weight control. You may even lose weight, depending on what your diet was before you started practicing yoga.

Yoga has been shown to be great at preventing joint and bone diseases like arthritis and osteoporosis. In general, when your joints aren't worked regularly, they often become inflamed, causing you pain later on. Practicing yoga puts you in positions that move your joints in ways they may not move during your day. This helps to release some of the fluid in the joints, thus reducing the likelihood of inflammation and arthritis. So yoga can help reduce your risk of arthritis. In the event that you currently have arthritis, work with your doctor to choose yoga styles that will help you instead of hinder you. Regarding your bone health, yoga is an exercise that uses weights to improve your muscle strength. The weight used is typically our body weight, but just like for those who lift weights, the weight strengthening the muscles also strengthens your bones. Stronger muscles tend to also lead to stronger bones. All of this can help reduce your risk for osteoporosis.

that placebo effect mentioned earlier, that when you practice yoga, you tend to ̣ a healthier life. A lot of people start to pay aᴛᴛᴇ_ ᴏn to their health, foods, activities, stress levels, etc. after practicing yoga. You may start to do the same with your yoga practice. All of this leads to a healthier outlook. After all, if you start to watch what you eat and what your activity levels are, you are more likely to make healthier decisions. You may start to go to yoga at least once a week, eat a bit healthier during the week, and maybe even go to bed on time. All of this leads to a cycle. What starts as just a belief of being healthier leads to realistic changes that make you healthier.

Beyond these physical aspects of yoga, yoga can also bring you emotional and spiritual well being. The meditative aspects, breathing exercises, and mindfulness associated with yoga can help you achieve a better emotional and spiritual state. This is especially useful to those who experience chronic illnesses. Yoga has been shown to help to enhance the quality of life for people who are diagnosed with cancer and other illnesses (Woodyard, 2011). So yoga can provide you with the means to have better wellbeing. It doesn't always lead you to healing because of yoga itself, but rather, yoga seems to teach people that they can heal themselves through their actions, thoughts, and behaviors.

Better flexibility

This should seem pretty obvious, but doing yoga regularly leads to better flexibility overall. When you first start your practice, you may have difficulty doing something like stretching your toes, or doing a side twist. But as time continues, you'll find that these poses become easier. The stretches associated with yoga help you to become more flexible over time, especially as you keep using those muscles. Since many aches and pains are associated with tight muscles, after practicing yoga you'll notice that previous aches and pains become few and far between.

This is especially helpful for senior citizens. As we get older, our muscles become tighter and we start to have more pain when moving. But yoga can help with this. In fact, in a study conducted with seniors who had regular aches and pains, the researchers found that after one year of yoga, practiced three times a week, flexibility was greatly increased in comparison to the control group (Farinatti, 2014). Having increased flexibility means that you'll have less pain in your joints and easier movements in your day to day activities.

Improved mental health

Depending on the type of yoga you use, yoga can be very relaxing. This of course, leads to feeling 'better' from whatever was bothering you. But even if you do a vigorous style of yoga, you can still receive the same benefits. Exercise in general helps you to relax, even if it's a pain to do it. Exercises like yoga help you to manage your body's stress response. They can activate your parasympathetic nervous system to help shift you into a more relaxed state. Thus, yoga gives you a feeling of relaxation which helps you reduce stress.

However, yoga also provides you with resilience. With that feeling of relaxation and by managing stress, your body becomes more resilient to future stressors. An aspect of this is based on how yoga reduces your cortisol levels overall. Cortisol is often fondly known as the stress hormone. With it's reduction, your stress levels will also reduce and remain lowered overall. This means that yoga can reduce your stress levels which can in turn improve your mental health. There are a significant number of studies that support yoga's impact on our stress levels and resilience (Link, 2017)

Yoga has also been found as a good exercise for relieving the symptoms of post-traumatic stress disorder (PTSD) and anxiety. In a couple of studies, women who practiced yoga and were also diagnosed with PTSD or anxiety were found to have significantly fewer symptoms of either disorder (Link, 2017). This could be related to the meditative aspects of the practice, since mindfulness and mediation have also been shown to reduce symptoms of anxiety and PTSD. The deep breathing associated with yoga might also help with both disorders.

Better physical fitness

Practicing yoga helps you increase your strength because the poses do require some strain. This strain helps you build some muscles. In fact, it's not uncommon to be sore the day after an intense yoga session. This is because of all the muscles you are using. You'll find that the poses become easier the more you practice them. This is because you are gaining the muscle strength to do them. The added strength and flexibility also help with your balance, which is critically important for seniors or those with health difficulties.

In a study conducted on the effectiveness of yoga for strength training, it was found that yoga did in fact improve muscle strength, especially after regular practice (Bhutkar et al., 2011). So with regular yoga activity, you can build on your strength and muscle mass.

Better emotional regulation

A couple of years ago there was a news article that came out and talked about how a school was using yoga as an alternative to detention. A lot of people thought this was crazy, but what yoga did was help children learn more about emotional regulation and prosocial skills, which was more than detention itself did. The school found fewer students having negative behavior and more students became interested in joining the yoga group.

This experiment in the school is backed by research. In 2015, a study was conducted with high-school students to see which helped them with emotional regulation and stability more, yoga or Physical Education. The results of the study found that students who were in yoga class gained significantly more control with emotional regulation and also learned more self-compassion and body awareness (Daly, 2015). Another study, this time with preschoolers, echoed this result with students gaining better self-regulation through yoga practice than through other interventions (Razza, 2013).

Thus, it's easy to see how yoga can be effective for helping children and teens work on their emotional regulation. It can also help them achieve more self-compassion, better self-esteem, improved attention in classes, and reduced behavioral issues.

Better self-image

When you go to a gym to exercise, you usually find a wall full of mirrors. This is, supposedly, supposed to help you with maintaining form in whichever exercise you choose. However, we all know that a part of it is vanity. We want to make sure we look good while working out and check ourselves (and sometimes others). However, in many yoga studios, you're not going to find mirrors. This is to help you focus more on yourself and your group and less on how you look while doing the poses. This can help with self-esteem and more body awareness. This can carry over into your day as well.

Yoga also helps with self-image because it generally helps you feel healthier and more satisfied with your body. It doesn't matter whether yoga helps you lose weight or if it makes you look better. You generally *feel* better after doing yoga and that contributes to better self-image.

Finally, yoga helps with mindfulness, as mentioned before. When practicing yoga, you're often in a mindful state. If you practice reaching that same state beyond your yoga practice, you're more likely to have a better self-image. After all, being mindful means that you're no longer focusing on the negative thoughts you might tell yourself. If you fail a test, being mindful means that you are aware of the negative thoughts, but you don't give in to them. Instead you focus on the reality of what happened and move forward.

Now that we've covered the basics of yoga itself, let's look into its rich history. While there is a lot of history associated with yoga, much of it is controversial since it's hard to keep records of something so ancient. Because of this, a lot of texts and manuscripts have to be interpreted and thus, the analysis differs from historian to historian. In the next several chapters, we'll cover what's known about yoga from 5000 BCE to modern days.

Chapter 2

Older Than You Think

Pre vedic era - 5000 BC

To understand the way that yoga developed through history, you must also know how history developed in the subcontinent of India. We're not going to go through an in depth explanation of culture or religion, but we will talk briefly about them. We're looking at a prehistoric civilization, that is so ancient, it isn't fully understood by historians. This era is called the Pre-Vedic Era, or the Harappan Era, based on the introduction of the Vedas in later millenia (the next chapter) or the site that was first discovered by archeologists. We are going to assume that this era started around 5000 BCE, since it's "official" start date is controversial and unknown.

It's important to note that the discoveries found about this civilization still baffle historians and archeologists. It's hard to point to clear indications of religious or cultural beliefs, but what is known for sure is that this was the time before a set religion. Many of the artifacts show that animals, plants, and nature were turned into deities and worshiped as such. Yoga wasn't even a thought during this time. However, the development of civilization during this era would begin the evolution of yoga. It would also set the stage for the development of Hinduism. Both yoga and Hinduism would develop together until they separate in later millenia.

During this era, the beliefs and understanding of nature and humanity were starting to be explored by philosophers and guru's. As each person or group started to explore their world, they set out to further understand how humanity fit in the wheel of nature. Some people focused on people in the world, and our impact on the world. Others focused on outside forces and how they affect the world. Another group focused on immortality and how life can be maintained. Others focused on how to be a part of the world without attachment to it. In essence to be free of it while also participating in it. Needless to say, there was a lot of exploration happening.

From these musings came important thoughts, and they were shared and passed through communities. Eventually, they were refined into sayings. It was believed that to get the true essence of what was being learned, you had to speak the knowledge in the same way that the original person did. So there was heavy emphasis on following set phrasing, pronunciation, and even tone. This led to the first mantras.

You are probably familiar with mantras. Our current understanding of them in the secular West is that mantras are something you repeat to yourself to further your own beliefs and goals. For example, if you are in a yoga class, your instructor might ask you to set your intention and repeat it as a mantra. A mantra might be something like, "I am beautiful and capable," to help you feel strong and confident during your day. While these mantras are definitely good and beneficial, they're watered down versions of the original purpose of mantras.

The original mantras were to impart universal knowledge so that humanity as a whole could advance. As these mantras developed, a key understanding of our 'self,' our inner being, and our soul also developed. Mantras grew to also include this metaphysical belief system.

It is from this belief that the first 'yogis' were born. In this case, yogis weren't what our modern understanding is. Instead, they were people who followed ascetic practices to further their own metaphysical beliefs and thoughts. Asceticism is the practice of removing a person from all worldly pleasure. A person who practices asceticism might choose not to eat, sleep, have sex, or engage in the world. But more often it's a more mild version of simply choosing not to have any worldly possessions or physical pleasure. All of this removal is to help the person reach more spiritual enlightenment. During this era and the era following, people who practiced asceticism were called yogins. And thus, the term yoga started to form into a belief based on spirituality.

But, like most things, the pre-vedic era came to an end. Historians aren't really sure why it came to an end, but their best guess is that the Aryan culture came and changed the prehistoric culture of the region. Their other guess is that new illnesses like leprosy and tuberculosis started to decimate the population. Either which way, the mantras of the time remained, as did their beliefs in the power of nature and animals. The pre-vedic era ended with the start of the Vedic era.

Chapter 3

The Rising Sun God

Vedic era - 1700 - 500 BC

Just like the era before it, the Vedic era is a little hard to pinpoint. The Vedic Era is marked by the first combination of the Vedas. Many scholars mark this as happening around 1700 BCE. However, other scholars argue that the Vedic texts were put together far before this. They mark the era as beginning millenia before, around 4500 BCE, so that's where we'll conclude that this era begins.

During this period of time, civilization was changing. The beliefs that would become the foundations of Hinduism were formed in this era. The word yoga also came into greater prominence during this era. The philosophy surrounding both Hinduism and yoga started with those mantras from the previous era and grew to be connected to the Vedas. The Vedas marked the first cohesive look at religion and spirituality, since it gathered all of the wisdom and mantras from earlier generations and put them together. They were the beginning of Hindu traditions and the beginning of moving away from the physical world to focusing on the internal one. These texts were further commented on by the Brahmana texts and Aranyaka texts. Because these texts were so instrumental in the development of yoga, these are the topics we'll explore in this chapter.

Vedas or Samhitas

Previously to this era, philosophers and wise people were exploring their understanding of themselves and their world. By this point, many people had started to understand the importance of keeping that knowledge. One of these people was Veda Vyasa. From modern day Pakistan and India, all of the wisdom of an ancient culture was gathered. Vyasa took it upon himself to collect the knowledge and wisdom of those who came before him and divide it into three books. When I say books, I don't mean literal books. During this time, the Vedas were still entirely oral, and weren't written down until much later, about 300 BCE. So Vyasa put organized all the mantras into three separate groups, to be told over and over again through spoken mantras.

The mantras put together in the *Vedas* became the basis of many religions in the area. What may even be surprising to some is how the wisdom within it echoes the wisdom in other cultures and nations during the same period of time. Even now, the *Vedas* are considered to be as highly regarded as the Bible in Western cultures. For something that has achieved such a high prominence, you might think that the *Vedas* were only about delicate philosophy of existentialism. However, that isn't the case. The mantras aren't focused on how to honor kings, or how to act and conduct yourself in ritual. Instead, they span to cover aspects of daily life all the way to metaphysical discussions.

Within the *Vedas*, you'll find text that cover how to properly farm, meet a good partner, or how to drive away evil spirits! It's a massive collection of wisdom. However, one of the key aspects of the *Vedas* is their discussion of philosophy. The *Vedas* discuss the importance of our inner and outer worlds and the connection between them. In particular, they discuss our human connection to nature and it's connection back to us. Some of the mantras emphasize the divinity within us, and others focus on the divinity outside of us. Either way, some of the philosophical aspects of the *Vedas* are about achieving a state of mindfulness to understand our connection to nature.

For those familiar with current mindfulness and mediation, might also be familiar with the belief that living in the past or the future puts us in a position of suffering, while living in the present gives us peace. This is something that was first started in the *Vedas*. In the *Vedas*, there are many hymns discussing our divinity and inner soul. The ignorance of our inner soul leads to misery, according to the *Vedas*. So they extol the virtues of learning about our inner worlds and connecting them to nature through mindfulness-like practices.

Because of this connection to mindfulness, many people believe that the *Vedas* are the beginning of a tradition of yoga. We'll get into this a little bit later. For now, remember how I said the *Vedas* was a collection of three books? Well there was actually a fourth, but this was added later on and not by Vyasa. Let's look into them because I promise at least one of them is connected to yoga.

Rig Veda

The first book of the *Vedas* is the Rig Veda. It's the oldest known Vedic text and was the first one put together. Rig Veda contains over 1,000 poems that are focused on divinity and enlightenment. Some of the people who contributed mantras were Vashishtha, a scholar, and Vishvamitra, a sage during the era. The hymns in the Rig Veda are used for praise of divinity. Because the hymns are focused on metaphysical issues, they are full of metaphors and analogies. One of these analogies introduces the term 'yoga' for the first time. This is the Dedication to the Rising Sun, hymn 5.81.1. Here's the translation, though in English, the word yoga is translated into 'yoke,' as that's what the word means, "yoke or joining."

"Men illumined yoke their mind and they yoke their thoughts to him who is illumination and largeness and clear perceiving. Knowing all phenomena he orders, sole, the Energies of sacrifice. Vast is the affirmation in all things of Savitri, the divine Creator." (Aurobindo, 1998)

Well that's totally easy to understand! Not really. Looking at this, we can kind of see how it's suggesting that those who join their minds with the enlightened sun, will also experience enlightenment and clear perception. Basically, this hymn talks more about a meditation with the goal towards clear perception. This is yoga, or yoking your mind to that of the sun.

That's very different from our modern understanding of yoga, but it does start the evolution in order to get there. Remember, our current understanding of yoga is a mix of physical exercise and mindfulness, so we can see how the Veda helps to start the meditative aspects of yoga.

The other Veda books

So the other Veda books don't really touch on yoga, but let's go through them really quick to complete your education on the *Vedas*.

The second book of the *Vedas* is the Sama Veda. This one contains chants, though most of the hymns have the same content as the Rig Veda. They're just written in a way so they can be chanted instead. What is quite amazing about the Sama Veda is that it's musicality has continued today, since it helped the evolution of Indian classical arts and created rules that are often still found in music.

The third book is the Yajur Veda. It talks about religious rituals and sacrifices and was used almost exclusively by priests. Like the Sama Veda, the Yajur Veda builds upon the Rig Veda. Yajur Veda is full of rituals that were followed during religious ceremonies, and are often focused on specific deities.

The final book is the Atharva Veda and it wasn't put together by Vyasa, as it was established much later than the other books, as already mentioned. It has prayers used for the average person and focuses on daily life activities. It also has a more magical style, as it contains charms for illnesses and incantations. It did also have some practices that led to later techniques of posture and breath retention, which were loosely related to yoga.

From the Rig Veda to the Atharva Veda, the philosophy within them start to change. The Rig Veda was all about the connection between man and nature and the importance of sustaining that connection. The Rig Veda most closely resembles the older religions of the previous era, with regards to divinity being everywhere and a focus on nature. But as the other books were added, they became more religious in nature, adding specific gods and rituals before ending the mythical folklore style of Atharva Veda.

During this period of time, the *Vedas* were used as a way of understanding and, to some extent, control nature and the cosmos. Rituals were critical for the success of this. However, as we all know, nature cannot be controlled. It will do as it likes. Because the *Vedas* say that rituals will control nature, many people were understandably angry when their rituals didn't work. Their anger toward the priests grew, and the priests realized they needed a better handle on the situation. The priests didn't want to admit to the fact that nature can't be controlled, so instead they blamed the rituals. According to them, the rituals weren't done precisely or accurately. To combat poorly made rituals and offerings, they created additional texts to add to the *Vedas*. This text was called the Brahmanas.

Brahmana Text

While the Vedic texts originally focused on the universality of life and the interconnection of humans and nature, the Brahmana additions started pulling away from this a bit, focusing instead on daily activities and practices that help people be more productive. They are not separate texts but instead added comments on the *Vedas*, written around 900 BCE.

The Brahmanas are extremely focused on refined rituals with the hope that the perfect ritual will lead to perfect results. This was the priests' solution to the anger of the people. If they could refine the rituals to incredible precision, then surely they'll work. So the rituals were all very specific. From the tone of a person's voice, to the shape of their hands, and the direction they're facing, all of this was carefully coordinated. So from the nature-human connection of the original *Vedas*, the Brahmana commentary narrowed it down to just the human aspect.

The Brahmana are a more worldly commentary on the *Vedas*. One aspect of the Brahmana is the focus on enjoying life while also contemplating a higher purpose. It's the first, basic introduction to ideas like karma, selfless action, and holistic health. These later develop into further aspects of yoga philosophy, Hinduism, and Buddhism. This focus on daily tasks and rituals continued throughout the late Vedic era. However, people became more and more against the rituals. After all, they were intense and required a lot. They also didn't always work. Thus, they developed another amendment to the Vedic texts called Aranyaka.

Aranyaka Text

The Aranyaka texts and commentaries mark a distinct change from the original *Vedas*. At this point, people are turning away from worldly pleasures and instead search for meaning elsewhere. The Aranyaka text focuses more on the inner world and our souls and minds, and less on the physical world. While there are still rituals involved, there is also a significant amount of philosophical work and soul searching. The Aranyaka often asked priests to go into the forest to meditate on their inner worlds and do their rituals away from the other villagers. The Aranyaka text was the start of the end of Vedic lore, with a strong connection to the *Upanishads* and the beginning of the Pre-classical era.

With the continued failure of trying to control the world, Vedic culture started moving away from worldliness and instead wanted to focus on their inner world. While they made this move, concepts like Karma and Dharma were starting to take root. From this change came new religions like Jainism and Buddhism. Both religions came and challenged Vedic beliefs by turning the eyes away from the world and toward the soul instead.

Jainism has a broad focus, with some focuses on understanding the many parts of reality and non-violence. It includes practices that aided in the development of meditative yoga. Buddhism, developed by the philosopher Buddha, also started focusing more on the soul and understanding reality as it is. It too has practices that lead to more of the philosophical aspects of yoga as we know it today. Finally, Hinduism, learning from these two religions, started adapting too.

During this era, a Yogin, or a person who studied the meditative qualities of the *Vedas* may have lived a very austere life. They would have abstained from most of the worldly pleasures around them in order to focus on their own spiritual growth. How they looked, dressed, and acted depended on how they practiced their beliefs. During the time of the Aranyaka texts, yogins would have lived in the wilderness, away from most civilization. They would teach those who came to them for wisdom, but would otherwise be separate from their physical world.

From this era, we can see the beginnings of yoga as a means for enlightenment, meditation, and focus. This era marks the beginning of an aspect that was essential to yoga philosophy, Hinduism, and other religions. The *Vedas* and their commentary started including aspects of a Supreme being, Universal Self, Supreme Consciousness, or true Reality. All of this referred to the understanding of being simply one part of a massive 'other.' That 'other' is described in many ways, but as the eras move on, it's sometimes called 'Brahma' in Hinduism, the "Universal Self" in Buddhism, or something else entirely. They all refer to the same aspect, the one overwhelming universal power. As we move through the next several eras, we will use all of these terms to explain some of the philosophy of yoga and its connection to that "other".

At this point, yoga isn't much. It's just a concept within a concept and hasn't yet been specifically developed. But during the next two eras, yoga will start to have more substantial development, before bursting into Western awareness.

Chapter 4

Where it All Began

Pre-Classical Era 500-200 BCE

This era marks the end of the Vedic era. During this time, there were massive changes to not only the civilization of the Indian subcontinent, but also a massive change in religious philosophy. There's a lot that could be covered in this era, but we will focus mostly on the religious aspects, since these are most closely related to the history of yoga. Again, we'll touch on a few of the texts of the era, and also look closely at Buddhism, which also contains relevance to the history of yoga.

The *Upanishads*

At the beginning of this era, the Vedic traditions were on the decline and people started turning to their inner worlds. The *Upanishads* were mostly written during this era, with a few before and after. Like the Brahmanas and Aranyaka texts before it, the *Upanishads* were amendments and comments to the *Vedas*. They are understood as the end of the *Vedas*.

The *Upanishads* are considered a foundational philosophy that impacted culture and the development of yoga. It is a collection of about 200 religious and philosophical texts, and currently, you can find and read about 100 of them. Unlike the previous religions before it, the *Upanishads* were about seeking internal, not external, spiritual quests. Some of them are attached to the Veda before, but many are not.

The *Upanishads* focused on helping people become enlightened. It's goal was to inspire people and lead them to the ultimate truth, rejecting blind faith, and accepting a universal consciousness. Some of the terms we still use today are based on the *Upanishads*. Ideas like karma and dharma are two principles that are echoed in modern variations of religion. Karma is that all actions have a consequence that is without judgement. The consequence is a positive or negative outcome and is the natural result of our actions. Dharma means having the right behavior, actions, and mindset. These two concepts are frequently found in Indian religions like Hinduism and Buddhism.

It is within the *Upanishads* that we come across the first definition of the term yoga. Of course, since the *Upanishads* were dedicated to controlling our minds to better understand the universe around us, the term yoga was mostly used to convey a mindful or meditative action, and less of a physical one.

In the Katha Upanishad, yoga is described as a yoke, or something that binds animals to a chariot. That doesn't sound similar to any aspects of yoga we understand now, so let me clarify. The Katha Upanishad used an analogy to help. Imagine an ancient chariot. Most chariots have two people, the charioteer and the rider, and two animals, usually horses. If a person can control the horses with the reins, then you can control where you are headed and reach a better place. Katha Upanishad explains that your body is the chariot. Your 'self' is the rider and your intellect is the charioteer. Your mind is the reins used to control the horses and your senses are the horses, able to determine objects on the path. So using this analogy, if your intellect and mind can control your senses, then you can reach a state where your senses are controlled and you become undistracted. This is the meditation of one's self, without the outside distractions. The Katha Upanishad called this yoga, the stillness of our senses and the focus of our minds. So for the philosophers writing the *Upanishads*, yoga was the meditative state that we can use to achieve a higher state of enlightenment.

The *Upanishads* also discussed another aspect of our modern understanding of yoga. The Prashna Upainshad talked about the breath and the energy connected to it. This energy, or life force, is called 'prana' in the Prashna Upanishad. The story of prana is amusing if you read it. It's basically a contest of which part of the body is better than the others, with the result being one winner.

The story goes that the five senses and prana were having an argument about which of them was the most valuable to humans. The eyes argue that without them, people cannot see where they are going, and humans would thus be injured. The ears say that without them, people would not be alerted to danger, and that they help humans listen to things the eyes can't see. The sense of smell piped in that they provide the richness of the world, and that while one can live without eyes and ears, that richness would be missed and so on. But when it was prana's turn, it said that without it, none of the other senses would exist to do what they must. The five senses didn't believe prana, so prana chose to leave to prove it's importance. As the senses became weak, they realized the truth, that without the life-force (prana), they were nothing. They apologized and the rest of the Prashna Upanishad talks more about the significance of prana.

Prana is the life force carried on our breaths. From this, the *Upanishads* introduced pranayama, or the practice of controlling the breath and thus controlling your life force. The goal of pranayama was to help calm the mind and control the storm within. This is an aspect of yoga that was key in the past. However now, pranayama is often overlooked. But during this era, pranayama was a key aspect of any yoga exercise. For people who focus on the spiritual aspects of modern yoga, the lesson of prana is often carried over into practice. With the energy riding the breath, current yoga practices rely on the breath to fill the whole body, thus providing that life force energy. By focusing on the breath and all aspects of the breath, prana can be added to our practice.

They also introduced the idea of pratyahara, or focusing on the self to the exclusion of the senses. This was also a key element of yoga during this era. It was a way to connect your outer self and inner self, and was a key component of meditation. It was considered the precursor to deep meditation since it required a person to withdraw from wrong senses and associations. This withdrawal leads to less distraction and better meditation, which is what yoga was during this era.

Thus, the *Upanishads* created some of the first known aspects of yoga. It added the meditative and breathing parts of yoga that we know now, though back then, yoga was still purely about reaching enlightenment.

Buddhism: The Middle Path

This era marked the beginning of the development of Buddhism. It was a philosophy that differed from the Vedas in that it rejected rituals, the priesthood, and sacrifices. Instead, it focused on our inner worlds and how that affects our outer world. Buddhism is called the middle path because while it does follow some ascetic practices, they are not supposed to be followed to the exclusion of the world. Instead, with Buddhism, the goal was to reach both meditative states while also still being a part of the world. This changed and adapted as Buddhism continued to be developed.

Buddhism is arguably the first time you get a systematic version of yoga. Of course, this yoga again focuses on meditation and the breath, but it also includes physical postures or behaviors to better support these activities. Buddhist text at the time supported this spiritual side to yoga. The postures were secondary to the meditative aspects themselves. There was also a psychological aspect of yoga in Buddhism, with specific techniques in order to rid the self of suffering and achieve enlightenment.

So as Buddhism developed, so too did yoga. It started adding more physical postures, reducing ascetic practices of wandering off into the woods to meditate, and added breathing and other exercises to improve yoga.

The Mahabharata and Bhagavad-Gita

Concurrent with all of this, the Sanskrit epic of *Mahabharata* was written. The *Mahabharata* is a story about violence and war. Unlike other epics like Beowolf, the *Mahabharata* doesn't encourage or deify war. Instead, it shows it for the devastation that it is. The victors of the war do not receive any happiness. In a few tales from the epic, those that receive happiness are those who practiced yoga and reversed their karma.

While the *Mahabharata* doesn't discuss yoga in particular, there are several stories that relate to yoga philosophy of the time. One of those stories is the tale of how a merchant met an ascetic. The ascetic, Jalali, practiced his beliefs by standing in the forest and meditating without food. He lived in nearly utter silence. He thought of himself as a very highly esteemed man for following his practices so well. But the gods told him that someone else, Tuladhara, was more highly esteemed. So Jalali went to talk with Tuladhara. Tuladhara, a merchant, knew all about Jalali and his practice. He rebuked Jalali for his pride.

So Jalali asks Tuladhara for advice on how to be more knowledgeable and moral. Tuladhara's advice was to act with nonviolence to every living thing, and to see all of the world's creatures as your equal. He advocated for the end of animal sacrifice and using animals for meat or burden. Jalali felt confused by this, and thought that this is wrong, but Tuladhara insisted that this is the true way to liberation. Essentially, the story talks about how spiritual values can be included in daily life. The practice of nonviolence was, at the time, practiced in Buddhism and Jainism and was thus introduced into Hinduism.

This story, and several others in the *Mahabharata*, emphasised several philosophical points like nonviolence, happiness in life, the reversal of karma, and vegetarianism, all towards the goal of reaching liberation and enlightenment. So how does this connect to yoga? Well, each of the stories regarding this topic help to show that meditative practices could help a lay person achieve happiness. These practices became part of yoga tradition. Before, ascetic practices used yoga as a way to achieve meditation by withdrawing fully from the world, like Jalali in the tale above. But the *Mahabharata* encourages the opposite instead. It encourages yoga practice where there is engagement in the world and holistic connection with nature. The lesson from these tales in the *Mahabharata* was that practicing these activities as a part of yoga would lead to a richer life.

By this point, yoga was starting to develop from a practice that removes oneself from the world, to a practice that requires you to be fully engaged. Only when someone was fully engaged in the world, could they enact positive change in it.

In alignment with this belief is the Bhagavad-Gita, a text that was first composed individually, and then attached to the *Mahabharata*. Like the *Mahabharata*, it tells a story with a complicated philosophical background. The Bhagavad-Gita is the story of a man, Arjuna and his discussion about war and death with the god, Krishna.

The Bhagavad-Gita is a story that demonstrates the connection between self and the universe. It emphasizes that yoga helps to achieve this connection (again remember, at this point in time, yoga was still spiritual in nature, not physical). It defined the purpose of yoga as connecting your individual soul with the universal soul, or Supreme Being, to become spiritually connected as one being. In the Bhagavad-Gita, Krishna represents the supreme being and Arjuna represents the individual soul.

The Bhagavad-Gita describes yoga and presents the first thorough discussion of yoga practices. It even tells you the goal of each individual practice and what you can achieve through yoga. According to the Bhagavad-Gita, there are 18 different ways to connect with the supreme being through yoga. Each chapter of the Bhagavad Gita explains how to connect better with the supreme. This is done through the 18 different yoga paths. They are:

- The Path of Dejection (Visada Yoga) - The individual struggle through life and seeking help beyond the material world.
- The Path of Analysis (Sankhya Yoga) - Using logical analysis to understand the universe.
- The Path of Action (Karma Yoga) - The natural consequences of our actions. Choosing actions that are service without attachment can lead to our freedom.
- The Path of Knowledge (Jnana Yoga) - Knowledge about the supreme being learned from a spiritual master, a yogin.
- The Path of Renunciation of Action (Karma-Vairagya Yoga) - Choosing to work for the supreme rather than just for oneself.
- The Path of Practice (Abhyasa Yoga) - Physical exercises that help to control the mind, body, and senses to connect to the supreme consciousness.
- The Path of Realization of the Ultimate Truth (Paramahamsa Vijnana Yoga) - Realizing the relationship between the material and spiritual.

- The Path of Imperishable Brahman (Aksara-Parabrahman Yoga) - The nature of living entities and death.
- The Path of Most Secrete Royal Knowledge (Raja-Vidya-Guhya Yoga) - Devotional service to the supreme.
- The Path of Manifestation of Opulence (Vibhuti-Vistara-Yoga) - Understanding how the supreme connects to the origin of everything.
- The Path of Vision of the Universal Form (Visvarupa-Darsana Yoga) - Knowing to find the supreme being within everything, and connecting with him through that knowledge.
- The Path of Devotion (Bhakti Yoga) - How to connect with loving relationships and devotion. It's the highest form of yoga.
- The Path of Fields and the Knower of the Fields (Ksetra-Ksetrajna Vibhaga Yoga) - How to connect with the supreme through enjoying life, nature, and consciousness.
- The Path of the Three Divisions of Modes (Gunatraya-Vibhaga Yoga) - We can transcend different emotional qualities to connect to the supreme being.
- The Path of the Supreme Enjoyer (Puru-sottama Yoga) - All living beings can learn to

enjoy life by working towards the enjoyment of the Supreme.

- The Path of the Divine and Demonic Qualities (Daivasura-Sampad-Vibhaga Yoga) - The qualities, both good and bad, of a yogi.
- The Path of the Three Divisions of Faith (Sraddhatraya-Vibhaga Yoga) - How goodness, passion, and ignorance relate to the supreme being.
- The Path of Advice for Liberation (Moksa-Opadesa Yoga) - Learning to work without attachment to the results of the work.

As we can see from these different paths, the concept of yoga is moving beyond just meditation to more specific actions and reactions. Bhakti Yoga is said to be the most important path because it connects loving action to the supreme being and gives the yogi the chance to fully explore and understand the universe. Essentially, the Bhagavad-Gita starts to show people how they can relate to the supreme while still being part of the world, instead of secluding themselves away from it.

If you're interested in learning more about the different spiritual paths offered in the Bhagavad-Gita, then I recommend reading it. In fact, it has influenced many aspects of Western culture. From our literature to our art, the Bhagavad-Gita has often been an inspiration point. Ralph Waldo Emerson even tried the different paths to yoga.

The Bhagavad-Gita and *Mahabharata* mark a significant shift in the understanding of yoga. This shift continues into the next era, with the end of the Vedic era and the beginning of the Classic era.

Chapter 5

It's a Classic

Classical Era 200 BCE- 500 CE

By the end of the Vedic era, yoga was changing from an ascetic meditative practice, to one that embodied a full philosophy on life and the world. Instead of focusing on removal from the world, it started to include belief systems that encouraged inclusion in the world. While the Bhagavad-Gita did provide the first explanation of yoga, this era produced definitive texts that still have a lasting influence on yoga practice. This chapter will discuss the influence of further philosophy on yoga's development and will introduce the first systematic form of yoga, Raja yoga.

The Yoga-Sutras

During the classical era, the writings of the previous era started to coalesce and develop. The *Vedas*, *Upanishads*, Bhagavad-Gita, and *Mahabharata* all started to create a distinctive philosophy for civilization. Among that was the emerging view of yoga. During the classical era, yoga is still mostly focused on meditation, but it also starts to take on a distinctive philosophy of its own. All of this came together in the Yoga-Sutras, a text that combined the wisdom of the previous eras into one, solid yoga philosophy. It was a text to help people achieve physical, mental, spiritual, and intellectual enlightenment.

The Yoga-Sutras were written or put together by a philosopher, Patanjali. While this single name may give you the impression of one writer, the truth is a little complicated. Many historians believe that the Yoga-Sutras were written over the course of centuries. That's a long life for one man. So it's more likely that the Yoga Sutras were written by multiple authors under the same name. Who ever wrote it, the Yoga Sutras provide one definitive explanation of Yoga, and it is still used today throughout modern yoga practice.

There are four main books and topics within the Yoga Sutras. They are the basics of yoga, how to attain the state of yoga, the benefits of practice, and freedom from suffering as a result of practice. These four topics help to organize the 195 sutras in the Yoga Sutras. The yoga sutras were written to help with meditation. It's full of knowledge on how to calm the mind so that it is focused. By following the sutras, it was understood that a person could achieve freedom from all mental and emotional suffering.

Within the Yoga-Sutra is an eight-limbed path to yoga, called Ashtanga. Yoga defined used all eight limbs, moving from the outside self to the inner self. The belief was that by using all limbs, a yogi could have a fulfilling life. The eight limbs are:

- Yamas
- Niyama
- Asana
- Pranayama
- Pratyahara
- Dharana
- Dhyana
- Samadhi

Yamas consist of ethical rules and actions. The focus here is about our own ethical standards and how we behave both externally and internally. They echo what was mentioned in the Bhagavad-Gita and *Mahabharata* in that the yamas call for non-violence to all living beings, truthfulness, non-stealing, fidelity, and non-attachment. In the Yamas, they explain actions for both internal and external beliefs. Nonviolence, for example, is connected not only to external nonviolence of others, but internal nonviolence too. So having nonviolent thoughts or words is a part of yamas. Again truth is both internal and external, with integrity being the internal aspect and honesty being the external.

Niyamas is all about good habits and self-discipline. They are often called observances because they are actions or rituals that you should follow. While they are practices to follow, they are based on themes, so there isn't a set ritual. The niyamas are purity or cleanliness, contentment and acceptance, perseverance, self-reflection, and contemplation of the supreme being. Just like with the Yamas, the Niyamas are for both internal and external actions. For example, purity and cleanliness can apply to things like your home and relationships, but it can also apply to your thoughts.

Asana is about physical postures, specifically postures that enhance meditation. There isn't a focus on poses. Instead, the focus is on postures that are comfortable and provide optimal alignment of the body. This alignment helps us maintain focus as we meditate. Remember that during this era, yoga is still focused on the meditative aspects, though we can already see that starting to change. The Asanas discussed in the Yoga Sutra are mostly seated poses, with the legs and arms positioned in different ways.

Pranayama is focused on the control of breathing. You may recognize this word, as it was previously used in the *Upanishads*. The idea is much the same. Pranayama is about regulating the breaths. There are various ways of regulating the breaths suggested in the Yoga-Sutras. Many of these are used today during meditation or mindfulness practices. The breathing exercises during modern yoga are our interpretation of basic pranayama. Pranayama is believed to help us focus on our meditation and rejuvenate the body.

Pratyahara is focused on withdrawing the senses. Again, this word may be familiar as again it was originally mentioned in the *Upanishads*. Pratyahara discusses how to turn the mind away from sensory experiences and instead focus on the inner self. This is the middle step, or the easing one to get the mind ready for meditation. It's important to distinguish pratyahara with asceticism. Pratyahara isn't about going into the forest or secluding yourself from people. It's simply about directing your mind's focus from the external to the internal while you meditate. It can also mean that you leave a space between action and reaction. This can mean that your mind is slightly distant and it gives you time to actually think before reacting. It's a hard skill to master, but one that is worthwhile. It's also the first step before going into meditation.

Dharana is about concentration and focus. It is the natural step that comes after Pratyahara as a person is now ready to focus more on the internal world, rather than the external. Dharana is focusing on one particular thing. It could be something like a mantra, a mental object, the breath, the body, a deity or even a thought. This is often what modern mindfulness uses, with the focus being on one thing and other thoughts passing by.

Dhyana is the meditative path. This path connects with the previous one, where you meditate on what was focused on. You start to reflect on it, consider it, and contemplate it. It is engaged, rather than passive, focus on the specific object of Dharana. The mind quiets the thoughts that are always buzzing and instead stays still, giving you the opportunity for peace.

Samadhi focuses on liberation. Liberation here means the liberation of the self. What was focused on becomes so in focus that the self is put aside.

Instead everything is combined into one. When in Samadhi, we are connected to the universal self and achieve great peace. This completes the path of yoga, resulting in ultimate fulfillment.

You may notice that these eight limbs progress in a specific pattern. They move from our external worlds to our internal ones. The Yamas and Niyamas focus on our behavior and actions. They focus on how we interact with society. The Asana and Pranayama bring the focus back to ourselves. The focus is on the body and the breath. Then we have the Pratyahara, which is our shift from the body to the mind. Finally Dharana, Dhyana, and Samadhi are entirely internal, with the mind focused on the self and the universal self. These eight paths take us all the way from society and people, to just us and the universe. It's an amazing path, and one that is difficult to complete.

As part of this path are the sutras, to help guide the yogi. The sutras themselves are very small. They're not like the epic of the *Mahabharata*, or the long story of the Bhagavad-Gita. Each sutra is instead like a small poem. They are typically not more than a few words. While they are small, they are powerful. The interpretation of each sutra can bring some enlightenment. It doesn't matter whether you are a beginner yogi or an advanced one, you can always learn from the sutras. To learn the sutras, it is best to have an experienced guide. Essentially, having a teacher can help you learn the deeper meanings behind the sutras and how to apply them to your life. Luckily, there are many interpretations available online, which can help you if you can't find a local teacher in your area.

While the sutras are complicated, their goal is worthy. By applying aspects of the sutras, a person could achieve a feeling of rest or focus. Everyday worries could be meditated on and set aside. Basically the goal was to improve our lives and help us connect with the universal energy.

Here is an example of a sutra from the Yoga-Sutras:

2.17 *drashtr-drshyayoh samyogo heya hetuh* (as cited in Holcombe, 2017)

We can see that this sutra is just a small amount of words, but the meaning is beautiful. Translated and interpreted, it ends up being:

"The cause of our suffering is the inability to distinguish between what is the truth (what perceives) and what appears to be the truth (what is perceived)." (Holcombe, 2017)

Wow, that is beautiful. What the sutra means here is that our inability to see the difference between what we understand and reality, leads to our suffering. But it can be further refined into understanding the difference between the Self and the Mind. The Self understands reality, but the Mind tries to interpret it to fit its own understanding. So we must understand the difference between the two and their roles. Only then can we have a clearer understanding, and reduce our suffering. That being said, another sutra explains that the suffering we experience can lead to greater clarity, so mistaking the Self and the Mind can lead to more understanding.

The Yoga-Sutras play a large role in our understanding of modern yoga. It is there that we can find and understand the more philosophical aspects of yoga, but it also started the movement towards postures during yoga practice. The Yoga Sutras created the first systematic yoga style, called Raja Yoga.

Raja Yoga is also called classical yoga. It is the original intended form of yoga, with a strong focus on the philosophical and spiritual aspects of yoga. It used all eight limbs of yoga from Patanjali's yoga sutras. If you are familiar with Buddhism, you might notice the similarity between the concepts of

Raja Yoga and Buddhism. This is because both developed in the same space, feeding off each other. While the Yoga Sutras are understood to pertain to Hinduism, there is also a connection to Buddhist philosophy. Buddhism influenced the Yoga Sutras, just as Hinduism influenced Buddhism.

Many of the lifestyle aspects of the Yoga Sutra is strongly similar to the lifestyle aspects of Buddhism. Both advocate for nonviolence and purity in thought and action. They also both call for care taken with others and society in general. For the meditative aspects, there is also similarity. The goals for both the Yoga Sutra and Buddhism are to find ways to alleviate suffering. They both call for deep meditation for this, as well as understanding the difference between Self and Mind.

Buddhist scholars developed their own work on Yogacara during this era. Yogacara was similar to the Yoga Sutras in that they helped to provide further understanding of yoga and meditation to the contemporaries of the time. It focused on reaching enlightenment through meditation and again understanding reality. So we can see that yoga was developing in relation to several different religions.

This era sets up yoga for the next millenia. However, the next era brings with it distinct changes to yoga and its practice.

Chapter 6

Less of the Mind, More of the Body

Post-classical Era 500 A.D.- 1700 A.D.

From the previous chapters, we can see that yoga developed into a richly philosophical practice. It was used to ease the suffering of yogis and focused almost entirely on meditation, with some suggestions for positions to better meditate. However, during this next era, things start to change for the philosophy of yoga. People start to take yoga and make their own versions, some of which are still used today. But, also significant, was the decline of yoga in India. We'll get into all of these aspects of yoga during this chapter.

Hinduism, Buddhism, and Jainism all influenced the growth and development of yoga in the previous millenia. They all developed together, so it makes sense that they also influenced one another. However, in this era they start to split from one another and create their own yoga styles. Some yoga styles were made as a split from Hinduism, while others were developed in Buddhism as it moved across the world.

In Hinduism, multiple new types of yoga were introduced in this era. Bhakti yoga, Karma yoga, Jnana yoga, Tantra yoga, and Hatha yoga all made significant changes to the yoga tradition during this era. These branches of yoga, all stemming from Raja yoga created a philosophy that was essential to Hinduism in this era. In Buddhism, yoga started making its name and also developed differently as Buddhism moved across Asia. In Tibet, Tantric Buddhism created Tantric yoga. In China, Zen Buddhism developed and maintained its own tradition of yoga. Many of these different styles developed within each religion.

For people of this era and time, yoga was a full time job. It was something that they practiced daily and often non-stop. It was their way to enlightenment and liberation from suffering.

Bhakti yoga

During this era, the Bhakti movement was moving across India. This movement marked a change for Hinduism. While Hinduism at this point did have multiple faces of god, Brahma, Bhakti focused on the emotional aspects of worship. Bhakti encouraged love and devotion to individual gods, one which you choose personally. In return, that god also gave the person the same love and devotion. There were different versions of the love between god and devotee. The relationship could be one similar to friends, child and parent, a servant and master, or lovers. It simply depended on where the movement was before the local population chose the relationship types that worked for them.

This movement developed across India very rapidly, resulting in changes to temples and worship style. These changes were echoed in poetry, art, and even buildings. It also changed yoga. If you remember from chapter 4, the Bhagavad-Gita explained how Bhakti yoga was the highest form of yoga as it focused on love for the self and the universe. In this era, Bhakti yoga was developed further, though it is thoroughly discussed in the Bhagavad-Gita.

Yoga was first considered to be meditation removing the world from the mind. Then it developed into connecting the self to reality. With Bhakti yoga, the connection changes again and becomes between the self and the universe or supreme being. It's a loving connection, flowing back and forth between the practitioner and the deity. In Bhakti yoga, the focus was entirely on that connection. There were songs, mantras, and poems used during yoga to establish that connection. Meditation was focused entirely on the divine. There were also rituals included. All of this was used to help understand the connection between the self and the 'Beloved' or the deity of choice.

Bhakti yoga and worship still has influence today, though many modern audiences change it to fit their own practice. Overall though, Bhakti yoga was one serious branch of yoga during this era.

Karma Yoga

Like Bhakti yoga before it, Karma yoga was originally mentioned in the Bhagavad-Gita, but it took several centuries before it was fleshed out into practice. Karma yoga focuses on selflessness and the importance of focusing on actions that result in positive consequences. In previous versions of yoga, liberation or enlightenment was reached through meditation or focusing on the divine. But in Karma yoga, enlightenment is reached through work, specifically selfless work.

However, there is a fine line. While the work in Karma yoga must be selfless, it can't be motivated by the consequences. So if you do actions on purpose because you know the consequences are always going to be in your favor, then that is not Karma yoga. Instead, the actions must come spontaneously without conscious consideration or thought. There must be no 'premediation' toward the actions. Basically, it's doing the best work you can without being attached to the consequences. The actions must be ethically minded without being biased towards one outcome.

As you can see from this explanation, there isn't any meditation involved. It is simply work. And yet, this is considered a type of yoga during this era. Karma yoga focuses on the service to others as your path to liberation. As a person continues to practice Karma yoga, it becomes easier, and the thought behind the actions goes away. Instead it is just automatic, resulting in personal development and connection to the universe.

Jnana yoga

Bhakti yoga is yoga of the heart and Karma yoga is the yoga of action. Jnana yoga is the yoga of knowledge. In Jnana yoga, the path to liberation is knowledge and wisdom. While this may immediately bring to mind someone studying in a library, or talking to a guru, this isn't the wisdom that Jnana yoga is about. During this era, Jnana yoga was still developing out of the yoga of previous millenia. What this means is that there was still a focus on knowing the difference between the self and the Supreme being. So Jnana yoga's search for wisdom was entirely connected to understanding the self and the universe.

In the other types of yoga explained in this chapter, the path to liberation and the end to suffering was thought to be achieved through love (Bhakti yoga), or kind actions (Karma yoga), and in Jnana yoga, that path is achieved through knowing the self. Knowing the self is more than knowing what we like or dislike. The knowledge of the self had to be connected to the knowledge of the universal self, so it disregarded thoughts like likes, dislikes, personality, etc. Essentially, Jnana yoga is about knowing our own minds and overcoming thoughts and ego.

Anything that is apart of our minds that can be modified is brushed aside. Instead, the focus of Jnana knowledge is to know the true essence of the self and the universal self.

From this description alone, you can tell that Jnana yoga is a difficult path. In fact, it's considered one of the most difficult forms of yoga, because to practice it, is to regularly strip yourself of all identity and focus on the self beneath it all. In Jnana yoga, the goal was to step back from our perceived reality to face true reality (like in other yoga forms) in order to know all 'selves' better. It's quite difficult, though still a worthy practice.

Within Jnana yoga developed the Sadhana Chatushtaya or The Four Pillars of Knowledge. These were aspects of Jnana that a yogi could explore to improve their practice. The four pillars are viveka, vairagya, shatsampat, and mumuk-shutva.

- Viveka focuses on discernment, or the ability to distinguish one thing from the other. In this case, it's the wisdom to distinguish between reality and thoughts, and the self and the universal self.

- Vairagya focuses on detachment. Just like in previous versions of yoga, this is about not being attached to things that are temporary. Things like ego and materials are considered temporary in this style of yoga. Knowledge comes from detachment. Jnana yoga encourages detachment from all things, even family, relationships, identity, etc. It asks for the practitioner to have a mind that is constantly in control.

- Shatsampat is called the six virtues that are used to stabilize emotions and the mind. The virtues are Shama, Dama, Uparati, Titiksha, Shraddha, and Samadhana. Shama is tranquility, or the ability to keep the mind calm. Dama is control, or the ability to resist the senses and use them only as instruments. Uparati is withdrawal, or the abandonment of activities that are beyond your duty. It calls for a simple lifestyle. Titiksha is endurance or the tolerance of situations that produce suffering. Shraddha is faith, or the belief in the yoga path. Finally, Samadhana is focus, or the precision of the mind.

- Mumukshutva focuses on yearning. It is the yearning to be released from suffering and achieving enlightenment. All other desires should be set aside. The knowledge of the self should be constantly engaged, firmly focused on being one with the universe.

All of these aspects of Jnana are difficult to practice. So Jnana yoga also includes practices for self-questioning and reflection. Meditation was still used during Jnana, but a practitioner was also encouraged to always use it, remaining in a state of awareness of the self and the universal self.

Hatha yoga

Hatha yoga is the yoga of movements and postures. While it utilizes postures as part of yoga, it's goal isn't the postures themselves. Instead, the goal is the movement of the prana. If you remember from earlier chapters, the idea of prana was established in an earlier era. Hatha yoga was developed to improve the movement of prana by using movements, the breath, cleansing, and hand gestures. Hatha yoga is considered to be a complete yoga path, combining physical wellness, mental discernment, and spiritual enlightenment.

Just as the other yogas were focused on the universal self, Hatha yoga was also about connecting the self to the universe. It was also about achieving balance in the self. It's said that Hatha yoga was meant to balance the masculin and feminine aspects with us. Essentially, it balances the mind and the body, transforming the body through the use of prana.

Within Hatha yoga there were several different steps and aspects. All of them were meant to help with meditation and the movement of prana. The parts of Hatha yoga are asana, pranayama, shatkarma, mudra, and bandha.

Asana is a set of postures. This is the most familiar aspect of yoga to modern readers. The positions in Hatha yoga are, in a little way, similar to the positions we take now during modern practice. Asana was the first step to help the body prepare for meditation. It was about controlling and disciplining the body. It was also used to remove diseases and illnesses from the body, while increasing the strength, steadiness, and lightness of the body.

Originally, there were only 15 postures associated with Asana. They weren't standing postures, but were mostly for sitting or laying down. These postures were to help start the meditation process. The original 15 postures were explained in the *Hatha Yoga Pradipika,* the first text with an explanation of Hatha yoga and Asanas. However, those descriptions were vague. Three centuries later, the *Gheranda Samhita* was written and it included 84 possible postures and positions, but mentioned that only 32 were for human use. So there weren't many specifics regarding the asanas for meditation.

The second aspect of Hatha yoga is pranayama. You'll, hopefully, remember that pranayama has made an appearance before. In Hatha yoga, pranayama was the method used to control the prana within the body and channel it through different containers in the body. Ideally, it cleansed the channels of the physical body and forced the prana into specific areas of the body. This was related, in some ways, to the beliefs on chakras which were developing during this era.

Pranayama consists of breathing exercises that helped to control the prana. The breathing exercises didn't have a particular method, but did encourage timing of breaths and the cessation of breaths. Later, pranayama techniques would develop that are often still used today. These include concepts like the Ujjayi breath, or Bhastrika breath. Both of these techniques were used to control prana and are often still used today in yoga practice. The breaths were said to cleanse the body.

The third part of Hatha yoga was shatkarma, or internal cleansing. The cleansing was considered necessary as a way to make room for prana's movements. There were six purifications; Dhauti, Basti, Neti, Trataka, Nauli, and Kapalabhati. Dhauti was the cleansing of the stomach. To do this, yogis would swallow a long piece of cloth soaked in water, and then remove it from the mouth. They would also use salt cleanses or air breathed into the digestive tract. Basti was cleansing of the colon. It was in essence an enema, with the yogi sitting over water and using their muscles to bring the water into their body through the rectum. Neti was a nasal cleanse. You might be familiar with that word as part of a "Neti-pot." Neti and neti pots rely on pouring warm liquid, or a warm thread through the nasal cavities, from one side to the other. Trataka was to cleanse the eyes, and required the practitioner to focus the eyes on a specific point (often a candle) until their eyes began to water. Nauli was an abdominal massage, using only the abdominal muscles to affect it. Finally Kapalabhati, which is a form of pranayama, was used to cleanse the chakras. This was done with forceful exhalations, with a strong push of air. The inhalations were slower, at a natural pace. The goal of all of these cleanses was to prevent illness and old age.

The final two aspects of Hatha yoga were Mudra and Bandha. Mudras were energy seals to move prana around, while Bandhas are energy locks, to keep prana in a specific area of the body. Each one contains positions for the body or hands, with contractions of specific muscle groups. If you have ever seen a picture of Buddha in his seated pose, with his hands in two opposite directions, this is a Mudra pose.

While each part of this sounds relatively simple, it was a very intense practice. Yogis would practice for years to get the positions, cleanses, breaths, and locks right. There were some that required extreme body modification, and there were many people during the era who were against Hatha yoga because of the physical aspects of it. However, it still remains one of the pillars of yoga during this era. In fact Hatha yoga is the yoga most frequently used in modern practice, though greatly adapted and changed.

Tantra yoga

Before we get into tantra yoga, I just want to quickly summarize the types of yoga already mentioned that were developed during this era. So Bhakti yoga was yoga of the heart and focused on strong emotional bonds with the Supreme being. Karma yoga was yoga of kind work, and focused on strong ethical duty. Jnana yoga was yoga of knowledge and wisdom. It focused on understanding the self and the ultimate self. Hatha yoga was the yoga of the body and mind. It focused on moving the life force through the body to maintain optimal health. All of these yoga styles were developed over the course of centuries and among them is tantra yoga.

Tantra yoga is both unique and the same. It is the yoga of ritual, but unlike the other forms of yoga, it isn't strongly connected with a specific movement or religion. Instead, it was all about understanding the mysteries of life and leaving the debates to others. It was also available to all people, not just the priests like some of these other forms of yoga were. While the other aspects of yoga were very philosophical, tantric yoga was more about practical application to help understand the relationship between humans and other forces. For tantric yogis, the goal wasn't to escape from suffering, but rather to live through every event, negative or positive. Finally, in the other schools of yoga, there was a belief that the spiritual world and the material world are separate. However, in Tantra yoga, the belief was that there were no separate worlds and they were in fact one in the same. So Tantra yoga has some very distinct differences in comparison to the other yoga types already mentioned.

Tantra yoga during this era was focused on ritual. While many modern people may understand Tantra yoga as pertaining to sex, in this era, Tantra yoga was about rituals including sacred sexuality. However, most of the practice has nothing to do with sexuality itself. Instead, it used ritual like mantras, deity worship, and mandalas, as well as a few similar practices to hatha yoga.

While Tantra was distinct from the other yoga types, it also gained a lot of traction in South East Asia, traveling very far. It influenced the development of many different religious sects, and was widely accepted by the public. While tantra was often associated with Hinduism, there was also a Tibetan Buddhist version called Vajrayana.

Like Hindu tantra, Buddhist tantra also used mandalas, chants, and other rituals. They also followed a similar philosophy, with the belief that the negative can be just as important as the positive in life. The understanding of each reality, both spiritual and material, is relevant, is also similar. However, it also connects more closely to Buddhist beliefs and paths, than to Hindu ones, with the goal of the practitioner becoming a Buddha.

So Tantric yoga provided a new style of yoga during this era that was markedly different from Raja yoga. All of these forms of yoga were passed on to learners through guru's or yogis.

The Life of a Yogi

During this era, yogis were becoming more revered as guru's or wisemen. They were the people you went to when you wanted to learn more about the connection between yourself and a greater power. Gurus were the ultimate wise people, already achieving spiritual enlightenment, and thus, worthy to learn from. There were often very strict aspects to each of these types of yoga, resulting in very distinctive yogis and gurus. Some gurus covered themselves in cremation ash, or never cut their hair. They may have stretched out parts of their body, or lived a life so frugal that they were incredibly thin. Overall, the guru's of the time who helped to spread yoga were very noticeable for the most part.

Yogis were not people who lived in temples. Occasionally, they would live in shrines, but often they lived alone in the wilderness. They would find homes in nature, by rivers or mountains. They lived off of what they found in nature, or what was given to them in offering.

If a guru was very popular, they would have a following of disciples. These disciples would learn from them, but also carry out their actions for them. It wasn't uncommon for disciples to go do the works of their chosen guru. From each guru came more styles of yoga and more disciples. Depending on the type of yoga they practiced, there could even have been religious monkhood as a part of the yoga tradition.

Most yogis were men during this era. In fact, there was a considerable reluctance and avoidance of having women being yogis. The exception to these were the practices of Tantra yoga and Bhakti yoga. Bhakti yoga encouraged all people to participate in it, and women were as equally encouraged as men. Much of Bhakti yoga became popular because of this inclusion. It didn't matter what gender or caste you were, you could practice Bhakti yoga. That being said, there were still some yoginis (female yogis) who were highly respected in other yoga traditions.

The Decline of Yoga

While yoga was growing and developing, it started to flourish in some communities and cultures. Unfortunately, India was hit with two major invasions that changed the way yoga was practiced. The first, was the invasions of the Mughals and the second was the invasion of the British.

The Mugal invasion did two things to yoga. In some cases, it suppressed aspects of yoga. Depending on who was ruling, Hinduism and other religions beyond Islam were often repressed, with wise men persecuted, temples destroyed, and other learnings prohibited. However, there were also rulers who were very tolerant of differences, and at least one Mughals warlord even learned and practiced yoga. The Mughals even influenced yoga in some cases, helping it's branches develop, especially with Bhakti yoga. By the end of the Mughal era, yoga was starting to decline but was still hanging on. However, that quickly changed with the invasion of the British.

I call it an invasion of the British, though I don't think many historians would quantify it like that.

However, let's be honest. The British invaded India and took over its culture, economy, politics, and society. With that came the crushing force of colonization, with aspects of Indian culture bent to shape European ideals. This included religion and language. One of the things to die under this reign was Hatha yoga.

Hatha yoga was already intense. It's physical aspects made some people wary and all of the physical rituals associated with it often made it a "sight to behold." After all, if someone can bend their feet behind their head, or spend their whole day balanced on the back of the neck with their feet in the air, this is something eye opening. It was also something highly confusing to the rational philosophy of the West. When yogis became poor under British rule, they often started to perform their yoga on the streets. The poses, repetitive actions, and the appearance of many yogis was visually disturbing to European audiences. Yoga quickly became synonymous with weirdness. People believed that Hatha yoga was off-putting, related to black magic, and basically reserved for the insane. In essence, it fell from favor hard and was brutally crushed by both the Indian people and the British. The British and the upper caste of India were all put off by the displays associated with poverty and yoga. The British instead encouraged other meditative practices that were less disturbing to their sensibilities, and yoga was put on the sidelines. This led to the rapid decline of yoga. It wasn't until yoga was introduced to the West in the next era that it made a resurgence.

Chapter 7

From East to West

Modern Era 1800 CE and onward

Yoga came to the attention of the West during the British colonization of India. But it wasn't until the mid 1800's that it was brought from India to Western countries. As mentioned before, at first Hatha yoga wasn't taken well, and yoga as a whole declined during the early part of this era. However, through the persistence of several different yogi's and Swami's (religious teachers), yoga came back. India was introduced to types of exercise that would influence yoga, and the West was introduced to yoga philosophy through multiple teachers. This chapter will talk about both sides and the development of the yoga we know today. The focus in these chapters is around the different teachers who influenced yoga and changed it from its ancient roots to a more modern version.

The 1800's

With the colonization of India, came the export of its goods, culture, and history. A part of this was the spread of manuscripts from India. This included the Bhagavad-Gita and other works. The Bhagavad-Gita was translated, sometimes well, sometimes not, and it started to increase the world's awareness on Indian culture. People became more interested in the philosophy behind the Bhagavad-Gita and wanted to apply that philosophy to their own lives. So they did. Authors like Henry David Thoreau and Ralph Waldo Emerson started to look to the Bhagavad-Gita as a source for enlightenment. Some of their works are based on their own meditative practice.

With the movement and translation of manuscripts came a new interest in yoga, in the West anyway. Europeans and American's hadn't seen the parts of yoga their counterparts found disturbing. All they were getting were the philosophical aspects from the manuscripts. To the Western audience, yoga presented a new type of spirituality, one that ended suffering and asked for kindness towards all living things. It was a massive change from the traditional religions of the time. At the same time, yoga was also considered to be something strange, uncouth, and depraved. People who had been to India had come back and told stories of the strangeness of yogis.

Because of this hate for many of the notable aspects of yoga like Hatha yoga, but an interest in the philosophy behind yoga, yoga made its way to the West in pieces. By the time the philosophical tenets of yoga made their way over to the West, they were changed. Many aspects of Raja yoga were set aside, and instead the more agreeable aspects were kept. Pranayama and meditation survived the trip to the West. Other parts like pratyahara, asana, and some of the yamas or niyamas did not.

During this evolution, came along a man who would be very influential for yoga in the West, but a little background first. A young man named Narendranath Datta spent a lot of his education learning about spirituality in the West and in India. He was a highly educated man, and like most highly educated people, he yearned to change the world, especially regarding social reforms in India. To that end, he took a very humanistic point of view in his philosophic learning and wanted to help enlighten people. He actively practiced Raja yoga and as part of his understanding of yoga, he knew he wanted to make society better. He wanted to spread education within his country, but also abroad. He believed that people from all religions could work together to achieve a better world.

Throughout his educational experience, he continued to be interested in spirituality. He was a part of several different sects, some of which advocated for an unformed god, and some of which worshiped a specific god. His whole outlook changed though, with his study with Ramakrishna. Ramakrishna was a guru in India during this era. From Ramakrishna, Narendranath continued to learn about the nature of spirituality and Hinduism. He learned to apply a kind of karma yoga, where he realized that service was the highest form of worship to god. He eventually became a monk and took the name Swami Vivekananda. He travelled across India and eventually Asia as a monk surviving on alms.

In the early 1890's, the first Parliament of Religions met in Chicago and there, representing Hinduism, was Swami Vivekananda. Originally, he had difficulty getting in as a presenter because he didn't have a certified background that people could confirm. After all, he was simply a travelling monk. However, he was finally able to get an invitation to the Parliament of Religions after receiving recommendations from a Professor at Harvard and another recommendation from a representative of his previous sect.

At the Parliament of Religions, Vivekananda gave several rousing speeches, discussing topics to do with Hinduism, Buddhism, Christianity in India, and the differences between religions. His speeches were short, but well accepted and respected. One topic of his speeches was his rejection of radical religion, and this included Hatha yoga as a part of Hinduism. Overall, he left a positive impression on the people from the parliament, so much so that he ended up touring a lot of the U.S., giving more speeches about the universality of religion.

By 1894, Vivekananada was settled in the U.S., and had started teaching yoga and Vedanta, or the study of the *Vedas* (yes, the same *Vedas* from 3000 years before). During his time in the West, Vivekananada worked to combine Indian and Western spirituality, adapting Hindu ideas to fit his Western followers. To that end, he taught his followers about yoga, specifically Raja yoga, Karma yoga, Jnana yoga, and Bhakti yoga.

He continued teaching, both in the West and the East. In the West, his focus was on spirituality, but in India, his focus was again social reform. He continued teaching yoga until his death in 1902. He left behind a legacy of yoga in the West and many disciples to follow in his footsteps.

While Swami Vivekananada helped to influence the start of yoga in the West, his work wasn't much different from the previously discussed forms of yoga. It was just adjusted to fit Western audiences better. However, in the next century, yoga would take a drastic change and become what we know today.

The 1900's

The 1900's brought a marked change to yoga. With information flowing back and forth between India and Western countries, yoga started to take a different shape. Through the 1900's different teachers of yoga started to influence how yoga would be used in the U.S. and the rest of the world. Some of the teachers included, Yogendra, Yogananda, and Krishnamacharya. We'll look at each of their philosophies that developed during this era, and also look at how they influenced yoga. But a quick note before that. There is something else that also influenced yoga during this time.

It makes sense that if things flow West, then they must also flow East. Exercise techniques from Europe started making a show around the world. They became incredibly popular and among them was a Scandinavian exercise called primitive gymnastics. Primitive gymnastics included the use of multiple poses to stretch and to gain flexibility and strength. It had such a far reach that it started to influence people in India too.

With the addition of primitive gymnastics to India, and other European sports and gymnastics, there came a fundamental shift in yoga. All of a sudden, the poses and positions from gymnastics were overlaid with the asanas in yoga. This lead to a massive significant change during the 1920's. Krishnamacharya was one of the first yoga teachers to connect primitive gymnastics and Hatha yoga, and it is that connection that we see in today's yoga practices.

Let's look at the different people who influenced the growth of yoga during this time.

Shri Yogendra

It's safe to say that without the work of Shri Yogendra, yoga wouldn't be what it is today. That sounds like a wide claim, but I guarantee that it's true. Yogendra's work was phenomenal and changed the way yoga was taught. His work with yoga helped lead to it's resurgence and led to a more modern version of yoga.

Shri Yogendra first learned yoga when he was in college. Before this, he had already excelled at physical activities like wrestling and gymnastics. He was very physically fit and well known for his abilities. But during his years at school, he slowly became more introspective and began to look for the meaning behind life. He met a yoga guru named Paramahamsa Madhavadasaji.

Madhavadasaji taught Yogendra about the power of yoga and its use for ending suffering. Yogendra learned how yoga could be applied internally, not just externally through asanas. For him and his guru, yoga was a way to heal the body and cure illnesses. To this end, he learned how to make asanas accessible for everyone to practice. He changed the form and the positions so that anyone could start learning Hatha yoga.

Before his work, Hatha yoga was just for those who lived separate from the world. But Yogendra encouraged all people to practice it. He believed that homeowners and households should learn Hatha yoga for wellbeing. He encouraged all people to participate, including women, something that wasn't widely accepted during this era.

Unlike previous yogis, Yogendra didn't focus on the spiritual aspects of yoga. He wanted to demystify it, and he was successful. It is because of his work that Hatha yoga rose up in the world and was seen in a more positive light. He helped to demystify yoga by looking for scientific evidence to support the use of yoga. He created the Yoga Institute in India, and later the U.S. to help research yoga and its effects on the body. He was able to find scientific support for yoga, which moved it away from a religious practice into more of a medical one.

At the Yoga Institute, Yogendra combined medicine and yoga, using it to heal the body. His work helped to establish the importance of health not being defined by an absence of illness. Instead, he defined health as wellbeing in all aspects of life. His life's work regarding yoga, philosophy, and medicine changed the game for yoga and made it more palatable for Western audiences.

You can see from his work here that he was incredibly influential. While yoga would have still developed without him, it was his scientific work that helped establish yoga as a means to wellbeing, instead of a means for spiritual growth.

Paramahansa Yogananda

One of the most influential figures for yoga was Paramahansa Yogananda. Because of him, the spiritual and meditative aspects of yoga are respected around the world. The spiritual focus wasn't new for Yogananda and throughout his life that's what he was looking for. He spent much of his childhood and teen years wanting to connect deeper with God and spirituality. He always felt connected to the spiritual parts of his religion, and because of this, he wanted to grow in spirituality. He looked for teachers among yogi's, guru's, and Swami's, and finally found a teacher he could learn from.

Yogananda worked with Swami Sri Yukteswar Giri, a yogi who was well regarded for his spirituality and teaching. He taught Yogananda about spirituality, social reform, and unity in religions. It was these beliefs that Yogananda took with him as he learned more about spirituality and yoga.

Like his teacher before him, Yogananda believed that all religions were actually one religion and that they were all the same, striving towards the same goal. He added this concept to his teachings and when he went to the U.S. for the first time in 1920, that's what he lectured on. He had many followers during his lectures and he became very influential and he eventually settled in the U.S.

During his time in the U.S., he created the Self-Realization Fellowship, which helped him develop his style of yoga. His work with yoga was strongly centered around meditation and became known as Kriya yoga. Kriya yoga is the yoga of action, and involves using mental states to control physiological ones. Yogananda taught Kriya yoga as it was taught to him by his mentor.

Beyond this, Yogananda published several books and articles. His schools for Kriya yoga furthered its interest. Through his disciples, and his schools around India and the U.S., yoga became more of an interesting topic for Western students. One of Yogananda's most famous work was his *Autobiography of a Yogi*. It was incredibly influential and many people have read it and been inspired by it. Even Steve Jobs. So I highly recommend you read it if you too want to be inspired by Yogananda.

Yogananda's yoga was very spiritual in nature. But our next influencers was physical in nature and led to the massive rise of yoga in the West.

Tirumalai Krishnamacharya

One of the most influential people that impacted modern yoga as we know it, was Tirumalai Krishnamacharya. He is often called the father of modern yoga and it is because of his work that yoga is what it is today. To be honest, not a lot is known about him because he never had bibliographies published, and didn't write as much about his life as other influential people of this era. He never left Southeast Asia, so whatever contact he had with the West was in his own home. What is known about him was passed down from his disciples, who spent years working with him, and his son and family. But each person has their own understanding of him, and some of their stories contradict one another. So here, we'll focus on some of the linking stories of his life and why he's known as the father of modern yoga.

From a very young age, Krishnamacharya was learning yoga. His father taught him the Yoga Sutras and other great works from when he was very small. The education at his father's feet resulted in a fascination with yoga that lasted a lifetime. But perhaps this also had to do with ancestry, since he was the descendant of Nathamuni, a yogi in the 9th century. Whatever the reason, Krishnamacharya became a lifelong learner of yoga and eventually a teacher.

Krishnamacharya was especially interested in Hatha yoga. Remember, during this era and right before it, Hatha yoga was still in decline. There weren't many people practicing it anymore. But Krishnamacharya was very much interested in it. He learned from the Hatha yoga texts and the asanas available. By the time he was 16, he had learned about 24 asanas, and he went on a search to learn more.

He told a story about how he started his journey about learning more yoga. Whether it's true or not, is hard to say. When he was about 16 he went to visit the shrine of his yogi ancestor, Nathamuni. There he had a vision. In the vision, an old man was waiting for him at the gate of the shrine. The old man pointed him towards a grove of mangoes and as he sat in the grove, he was surrounded by three yogis, all venerable men. One of them was his ancestor, Nathamuni. He prostrated himself before them and begged them to teach him about yoga. For hours, they did. They gave him instructions on yoga and called it the contents of the *Yogarahasya,* a text on yoga that hadn't been seen for well over a millenia. Being a faithful student, Krishnamacharya wrote down all that he learned from those yogis. He used the knowledge to spur him on his quest to know yoga. If you're interested, you can actually read the text that he recorded. It has been translated and is available to purchase.

From that one vision, Krishnamacharya chose to continue his path to learning yoga. He found instructors and along the way he found a Hatha yoga master, Ramamohan Brachmachari. There isn't a lot known about Brachmachari, other than he was a yogi who lived in the mountains. He supposedly knew over 7,000 asanas, which was a feat since the previous texts on Hatha yoga only spoke about 84 of them. Krishnamacharya made the long journey to see Brachmachari and studied with him for nearly eight years. During his study, he learned more about hatha yoga, yoga in general, and multiple asanas and pranayamas. After his work with Brachmachari, Krishnamacharya left the mountains to teach yoga.

He taught yoga to everyone who would listen. He walked around from place to place giving lectures and demonstrations. To him, the only way to spread the teachings of yoga was to show what it could do. So he used amazing demonstrations that showed what yoga could do for a person. Some of these demonstrations included doing difficult asanas, or showing feats of strength. With each demonstration, the interest in yoga grew. When he was finally given a space to teach, his students were in fact people who witnessed his demonstrations.

At the college he was hired to teach at, Krishnama-charya gave continued lectures on yoga and other philosophy. By this point, he was well educated and had a good knowledge of many of the classical Indian disciplines like rituals, law, logic, and medicine. With all of this background, much of what he taught about yoga pertained to how yoga could heal and increase well being. When he started teaching yoga asanas themselves, it was with these goals in mind.

Krishnamacharya knew that the original Hatha yoga asanas were unpopular. So he created a new style of yoga. He combined the original asanas with scandinavian gymnastics techniques. By this point, primitive gymnastics, a style of Scandinavian gymnastics became wildly popular around the world. In the poses and positions, there were great feats of flexibility and strength. They also tended to flow well together. Krishnamacharya took this style of gymnastics and combined it with traditional asanas, pranayamas, and meditation. He then developed flowing asana techniques, a style now known as Viniyoga.

He knew that the asana sequences were difficult and he really pushed his students to do well. So he divided the sequences by ability type. Beginners, intermediate, and advanced level students each had their own flowing asanas. They were hard, and he was a brutal taskmaster, asking his disciples to work through difficult positions.

During this period of time, he gained many students. These students helped spread his work to the west and other areas. We'll talk about his students in a little bit.

In 1947, India got its independence from Britain. It changed the social and political sphere that

Krishnamacharya normally worked in, and he faded a bit into obscurity. However, his work never ended. Because he knew that yoga couldn't be sustained for everyone, he learned to adapt his yoga to people of different abilities. For him, yoga became a method of healing the sick, so he started working more with children, the elderly, and the ill. He even started working with pregnant women to help them during the pregnancy. Remember, he had a background in medicine that also backed up his yoga practice. His new form of yoga moved away from the difficult asanas of his previous teaching, into ones that were more supportive and helpful for the wellbeing of the practitioner. From this growth, he realized that his yoga style could again be divided. The yoga of his previous years was reserved for youth, because of its focus on strength, power, and flexibility. For health and vitality, he changed his yoga style for those in their middle ages. Finally, he put together meditative practices for those in old age as their form of yoga. His style of yoga didn't really have a set name, but it influenced Vinyasa, Ashtanag, and Viniyoga.

He continued practicing and teaching yoga until his death at age 100. His yoga practice was always a combination of asanas, pranayamas, and meditation and had been so successfully adapted that anyone, young or old, fit or not could practice it. Krishnamacharya is well known in India as a scholar and healer, and less of a yogi, since his yoga practice was mostly for healing.

Tirumalai Krishnamacharya was called the father of modern yoga for a good reason. It's because of him that yoga has become what we know today. It's also his work that helped with the resurgence of yoga in India. His life and work influenced many students, including Pattabhi Jois, B.K.S. Iyengar, Indra Devi, and T.K.V. Desikachar, all of whom later went to develop their own forms of yoga. They took his lessons and applied them to their own yoga forms. These four (and many other) disciples of Krishnamacharya can be credited with spreading yoga in the West. Their works have honestly led to what we now call modern yoga.

We will get into these different types of yoga in the next chapter, but I want to briefly touch on each of the people who worked under Krishnamacharya to spread yoga around the world:

- Pattabhi Jois studied under Krishnamacharya for 22 years. During that time, he learned a lot from Krishnamacharya. When he left, he used the yoga he learned from Krishnamacharya to develop yoga further.

He didn't change what was taught to him, but he did refine it. He created Ashtanga Vinyasa Yoga, now known as Power Yoga.

- B.K.S. Iyengar was another student of Krishnamacharya. He was sickly but studied under Krishnamacharya to improve his health and wellbeing. He only studied under for a year, but it was an influential year. Iyengar took from Krishnamacharya the healing aspects of yoga. He then created a yoga style that helps people from all walks of life by using props. His form of yoga works a lot on healing and wellbeing beyond the other aspects of yoga, and it led to considerable research about the healing aspects of yoga. He created Iyengar Yoga, which is still offered today and widely used.

- Indra Devi broke the mould for Krishnamacharya because she was probably his first female student. He taught her rather reluctantly, but still taught her his version of yoga. However, he changed it a bit. Unlike with his other students, Krishnamacharya did not use harsh techniques but used a gentler approach when working with Devi. This gentler approach is echoed in her own practice and teaching. Once she moved to the U.S., Devi started teaching yoga to celebrities and marketed her yoga as one for women as a remedy for stress. Her work with celebrities helped spread the popularity of yoga in the U.S. Her focus on gentler yoga for women can be credited with the spread of yoga as a feminine exercise, though we of course now use it for all genders. Devi focused mostly on asanas, pranayamas, and some meditation, though she didn't include the spiritual aspects of yoga her fellow classmates did. The style of yoga that Devi taught is gentler than our current forms of yoga, but can be similar to slower Hatha yoga practices.

- T.K.V. Desikachar is the final pupil that we'll discuss. Desikachar was the son of Krishnamacharya and he learned yoga from his father, just as his father did from his grandfather. With Desikachar though, there wasn't a lot of practice from a young age. He apparently detested yoga until he learned about how it helped heal people and bring about their wellbeing. It was then that he became interested in knowing more about yoga. Learning about yoga from his father also helped him become a good teacher. Unlike his father, Desikachar wasn't religious and didn't believe in the mysticism related to yoga, so his own areas of focus as a teacher were on wellness, not on spirituality. He published many books on yoga and developed Viniyoga.

So you can see from Krishnamacharya's teachings we have the branches that started yoga traditions in the West. Some people say that nearly every modern version of yoga is, in some way, connected to Krishnamacharya and his yoga style. They would probably be correct and most versions of Western yoga are related to the Hatha yoga style that Krishnamacharya helped establish. Krishnamacharya's adaptation of Hatha yoga changed yoga from a practice that was mostly spiritual, to one that was mostly physical. It is this physicality that is represented throughout modern yoga practices.

Today

The influential work of these three men and their disciples led to a renaissance of yoga. In both the West and India, yoga became more popular and was regularly practiced. Today, most yoga is physical, following the style of Krishnamacharya. Hatha yoga has become synonymous with yoga now. If you are taking a yoga class, it's most likely going to be a Hatha yoga class, even if it's called something like Vinyasa. These classes are simply the most common as the focus during today's era is on physicality instead of spirituality. That being said, there are still many schools of Kriya yoga and other spiritual yoga classes available.

Yoga went from near extinction during the British colonial period to great resurgence. In the U.S., nearly 36 million Americans have practiced yoga. The number of people who practiced yoga drastically increased over 50% in a four year period alone. Today, many practitioners are women. In fact most are, which is a huge difference from the ancient practice of yoga.

If you were to go out today to join a yoga class, you are most likely going to find one that is physical only, full of asanas and occasional pranayamas. However, if you live in a larger city, you'll likely find yoga classes that work with all aspects of yoga, even the ancient versions. Yoga is no longer something practiced by forest dwelling yogis. Instead, it's practiced by everyday people, and enjoyed everywhere, including gyms, parks, homes, and schools. It's a massive difference in just under 7000 years of yoga.

Today, yoga is understood as a mindful physical exercise based on several guiding philosophical principles.

- The first principle is about the human body. Each aspect of our bodies are interconnected and one part affects the others. Our bodies can also heal ourselves through movement or rest.

- The second principle is that we are all uniques. Our needs and our 'selves' are unique and so our yoga practices must be adjusted to fit our needs. Krishnamacharya and others started the process of adapting yoga to fit everyone's needs and today you can find classes that fit you. Fully trained teachers can support their student's needs with yoga, no matter what those needs are.

- The third principle is that yoga is empower-ing. Yoga can lead you to improve your own life and healing yourself. It actively helps you understand that healing comes from within you. This is an ideal that was echoed in the teachings of all of the modern yogis. Yoga was always about self empowerment and development.

- The fourth principle is that our minds are crucial for our growth and health. When we have a positive mindset, we can grow and heal ourselves. Again, this is a pattern that is echoed in yoga throughout the centuries. The Yoga Sutras and other writings all emphasize the importance of the mind and knowing our thoughts in order to grow.

There is another change in today's version of yoga. Before, yoga was the purview of mostly men, and mostly men who were followed by disciples. While there are some gurus today who also have disciples, most of this has been changed to teachers who train others to teach. There isn't discipleship in particular, at least not in the way of the past.

Another change is also about who could practice. In past yoga tradition, yoga was mostly for men. Today though, most yoga practitioners are women and it has spread as a more female-centric practice. Many of the yoga types that are established now were established by women. So there was a serious shift in that aspect of yoga.

The other shift was in body type and care. Yoga today is for everyone. It doesn't matter whether you are injured, have a disability, are plus-sized, are thin, or are fit. Yoga can be for you. In previous era's yoga was mostly for people who were able bodied and practitioners were often very thin, probably due to the lifestyle differences. This change in yoga is very positive as there is now more inclusion within yoga practices.

So there you have it. Yoga's development from 5000 BCE to 2019 CE. It's come a long way and changed to fit the world as it was needed. In the next chapters, we'll discuss some of the different styles of yoga found today. We'll also discuss the modern connection between religion and yoga.

Chapter 8

From One Came Many

In the last chapter, new modern styles of yoga were introduced, though they weren't thoroughly discussed. This is the chapter where we'll explore the different kinds of yoga that are practiced today. Out of the original styles of yoga, Bhakti, Karma, Jnana, Hatha, and Tantra, there are now a multitude of different styles of classes taught. It's easy to find one to fit your needs, whether they are spiritual, mental, or physical needs.

As you go through the chapter, consider which types you would enjoy, and keep in mind that just because a practice is physical, doesn't mean it can't be spiritual for you too, if that's what you're looking for. Whether you are currently practicing, want to practice in the future, or will never practice but want to learn more, this chapter will set you up for understanding the key facts of the many yoga classes out there.

Before we get started going through these kinds of yoga, make sure that you are familiar with the yoga terms in chapters 5 and 6 as many of these terms are used to describe these classes. To help you remember the basics:

- Asanas are postures or positions for yoga. In our modern practice, asanas are a mix of standing, lying, and seated positions, with a few headstands and shoulder stands thrown in.
- Pranayama are breathing techniques used during yoga practice or meditation. It is about controlling the breath. Many pranayama practices you'll hear in your classes include the Ujjayi breath (where the breath makes a sound as you inhale and exhale) and the Bellows breath (where the air is forcibly exhaled).

Today, you're very likely to come across classes simply titled Hatha yoga. These classes are not like the Hatha yoga of old, but are usually a mix of yoga styles. You'll have activities with asanas and perhaps some pranayama, but other aspects of yoga may not be included. To find out more about what the class will involve, talk to the teacher and check with their training. Their training will influence the style of the class. Typically, classes labeled as Hatha yoga are classes where positions are held for a bit before moving to the next position. They are a slower flow of yoga. However, this may not be the case with all Hatha yoga classes.

Yoga for a Workout

If you are looking for a yoga practice that is mostly physical in nature, then these are the ones you want to try. These yoga types usually include asanas and pranayamas. Occasionally, they'll include other aspects of yoga, but these are mostly used to increase your strength and flexibility. They are a workout. This means that you need to be prepared to really exercise when you're in these classes. These classes are not for people who are new to exercise or who have injuries. You will get a great cardiovascular workout from these classes, so be prepared for your heart to race.

Vinyasa style yoga is based off the teachings of Tirumalai Krishnamacharya. It is a yoga that goes through a series of positions and movements quickly, with an emphasis on flowing from one pose to another. It's very intense and will cause you to sweat as you practice it. From Vinyasa came Ashtanga.

Ashtanga was created by Krishnamacharya's pupil, Pattabhi Jois. Just like Vinyasa, it's a very intense version of yoga. There are set sequences that are repeated over and over again, going from simple positions to harder ones. It's not a yoga style where you can pause between positions to adjust. You keep moving and it is very physical, which can be a perfect option if you are looking for a cardiovascular workout or strength building. Ashtanga does have some breathing emphasis, but not a lot. During your class, you'll be told when to breathe to help you flow through the movements quickly. Your movements will follow the breath. Ashtanga is done at your own pace. You'll learn the asanas and the sequences but then you'll follow the practice at your pace. It's a good idea to be familiar with the sequences and to practice them at home so that you can follow the class well.

Power yoga is another form of Vinyasa yoga. This was created by Bender Birch, in 1995. Power yoga is very similar to Ashtanga in that it's very physical and will give you a workout. However, it doesn't follow the same patterns of Ashtanga. It also focuses almost solely on asana instead of other parts of yoga. It keeps you constantly on the move and gives you a very good strength workout. You have to be in physically good shape when practicing power yoga as it is not for people who are just starting to workout. It's too intense for someone who hasn't already been exercising regularly.

Bikram yoga was created by Bikram Choudhury. It's a style of yoga that is very different from these other kinds and it is often called "hot yoga." This is because you'll get very hot while practicing and I don't mean that you'll get hot from the workout alone. Bikram yoga is held in a sauna like environment, with temperatures as high as a humid summer's day in Florida. The purpose of Bikram yoga is to cleanse the body through asanas and sweat. If you choose to practice Bikram yoga, you want to make sure that you are very hydrated and are okay in hot environments. The asanas in Bikram yoga are a mix of standing poses and floor poses mixed with pranayama. Every class uses the same asanas and pranayamas. The teachers also follow the same pattern, so once you know each part you're set in the class.

Well Balanced Practices

If you want a yoga style that incorporates asanas, pranayamas, and meditation, among others, then these are the classes you want to look for. Many of these classes are only offered in very specific locations, but you can find the nearest one to you by looking at their respective websites.

White Lotus yoga was developed by Ganga White and Tracey Rich. This style of yoga is similar to vinyasa in that it has flowing postures. However, these movements have a variety of skill levels and each class incorporates other aspects of yoga, including theory and pranayama. White Lotus yoga is offered at specific retreats.

Kali Ray TriYoga was developed by Kali Ray in 1980. This yoga style uses asanas that are similar to dancing poses. Unlike some of the other yoga types, this class includes music and more focus on each movement during a sequence. It combines the use of asanas, pranayamas, meditation, and mudras. To help remind you, mudras were discussed in chapter 6 on Hatha yoga and are a way to move prana in the body through specific body movements. In TriYoga, mudras are used through hand gestures. TriYoga is a way to fully experience yoga and have both an outer flow through the postures, and an inner flow.

Jivamukti yoga was created by David Life and

Sharon Gannon in 1986. It is just as physical as Ashtanga, but includes more meditative practices. In fact, you might consider it to be very similar to Raja yoga, just interpreted for our time. It shares some of the same philosophy behind it. The asanas are still there, but mediations are incorporated into the class. A Jivamukti class will also include lessons on chanting, and sometimes review some key yoga texts. It also encourages specific lifestyle changes, similar to the yamas and niyamas of previous styles of yoga. It's a class for a fully rounded style of yoga.

Physically Supportive Yoga

If you are looking for a style of yoga that is physically supportive, then these are the kinds you want to look for. These styles of yoga are perfect if you want to use yoga as therapy or for healing. They're also great if you want yoga classes that are precise and adaptable to the needs of every participant.

Integrative Yoga Therapy was developed in 1993 by Joseph Le Page. This style of yoga is more medical in nature, helping participants heal. It is a yoga that is gentler in nature and is used in many medical facilities around the world to help support people struggling with diseases and disorders. It incorporates some asanas as well as pranayamas, and guided imagery meditation. The reason why Integrative Yoga Therapy is included in this section instead of the previous one is because it is meant as a supportive yoga, and not necessarily a spiritual one, though you can use it as that if you like. It is a very student-centered practice. This means that it is adapted to each student's needs and takes their abilities into consideration.

Iyengar yoga was developed by B.K.S. Iyengar, a disciple of Krishnamacharya. It is strongly connected to the Yoga Sutras, despite being also connected to Krishnamacharya's Hatha yoga. Iyengar yoga focuses on the physical alignment of each posture and breathing within each posture. So each position is held for several breaths while the focus is on the muscle, joint, and bone alignment. You'll only do a couple of asanas in the class, since the focus is on the minute movements of your body. Iyengar yoga is different from other types of yoga because it uses a variety of props to help physically support the practitioners. It's not uncommon for blocks, towels, belts, and chairs to be used during the practice. Because it includes so much support, Iyengar yoga is a great class if you have concerns about your abilities. It can be adapted to people of all abilities and injuries. Iyengar yoga is probably one of the most popular forms of yoga in the world and is perfect for beginners.

Phoenix Rising Yoga Therapy is a mix of yoga and psychotherapy. Like other styles of psycho-therapy, Phoenix Rising is about establishing a therapeutic relationship with the teacher and using that to heal mental, physical, emotional, and spiritual difficulties. The style of yoga is similar to Raja yoga and the postures are assisted. It uses asanas, pranayamas, and conversation to elicit change.

Viniyoga is another holdover from the teachings of Krishnamacharya. Viniyoga was developed by his son, T.K.V Desikachar. This form of yoga is considered to be more gentle than it's other counterparts. It focuses on asanas, pranayamas, meditation, and good health. To that end, Viniyoga is highly supportive. Each class is catered to it's participants and the sequences are adapted to fit everyone's ability. Viniyoga is considered to be very adaptive to help people reach their goal of good health. The teachers will literally go around and make modifications for each student as necessary. Because of this, Viniyoga is perfect if you are working on pain management, are a senior, or have a disability. Viniyoga will fit your needs.

Spiritual Yoga

If you are looking for a yoga class that is more reminiscent of yoga in the past, then these are the classes for you. Many of these classes are not only about asanas and pranayamas, but they usually also contain a spiritual focus and a community one. These are yoga classes that encourage lifestyle changes and you should consider using them in a daily way. They will help you grow, both in strength and flexibility, but they'll also help you grow spiritually, to better understand your 'self.' My personal favorite is Kundalini, however, it can be difficult to transition into for beginner yogis.

Integral yoga was introduced in 1966 by Reverend Sri Swami Satchidananda. It is a philosophy based yoga, reminiscent of past yogas. In fact, it is praised as a style of yoga that is close to the original purpose of yoga. It combines karma yoga, bhakti yoga, jnana yoga, and hatha yoga. It was created so that people could use it everyday. The spiritual aspects of this style of yoga are based on wanting to make the world a better place. So the goal of this style of yoga is to help people achieve peace and spread that out into the world. Integral yoga is a very meditative yoga practice. Each movement is part of meditation, with pranayamas, mantras, chants, and guided relaxation included in the class.

Sivananda yoga was introduced to the U.S. in 1957 by Swami Vishnu devananda. This style of yoga is focused on understanding the self. It incorporates aspects of Bhakti and Karma yoga to help the practitioner develop their spiritual selves. Sivananda combines aspects of your life, like diet and positive thinking with meditation, asanas, pranayama, and savasana (relaxation). Unlike other yoga styles that use multiple different postures, Sivananda uses only 12 basic postures.

Anusara yoga is a style of yoga that combines movement with spiritual awakening. It combines Hatha yoga asanas with affirmations and meditation, to combine body, mind, and spirit. It is based on tantra yoga philosophy and many of its practices follow those same ideals. There is a strong community focus, with the goal of supporting students in all aspects of their life.

Kundalini yoga was introduced in 1969. It is based on tantra yoga and the belief that there is energy based in the spine (Kundalini). Each movement, posture, breath, and meditation is used to move that energy up through the chakras of the body. Kundalini uses many aspects of traditional yoga, like asanas, pranayamas (with specific focus), and mudras, among others. Pranayama is especially used in Kundalini, as there are several challenging breathing exercises that it uses. It's a very spiritual form of yoga while also being a very physically challenging one. Kundalini yoga is unique in that many practitioners wear specific garb and clothing (mostly in white) during practice. There is also a focus on early morning practices and other lifestyle changes. The classes are usually a good mix of asanas, pranayamas, and meditation

Ananda yoga was developed in the 1960s by Swami Kriyananda. He learned under Paramhansa Yogananda who taught Kriya yoga and Karma yoga. While Ananda yoga uses postures, breathing, and meditations, it also uses quiet affirmations during each pose. This helps to deepen the purpose of each pose. It's a gentler yoga than power yoga and it reflects an older style of yoga. Each pose is there to help prepare the practitioner for meditation. The whole purpose is spiritual growth through each movement and breath. If you remember from previous chapters, this is very similar to the classical styles of yoga.

Integrated Science of Hatha, Tantra, and Ayurveda (ISHTA) yoga is, as the name suggests, a combination of different styles of yoga and medicine. Ayurveda is a traditional medicine that is practiced in India. The goal of the classes is to get participants in touch with their prana and senses. It combines vinyasa flowing asana with pranayama, and meditation. It also includes some cleansing techniques. All of this is done to balance the human body and its energy.

Tibetan yoga is a form of yoga that is based on tantric yoga from Buddhism. It is an active form of yoga, that revolves around sequences of asanas. These asanas are repeated multiple times during practice. However, like the tantra yoga of older times, there is a strong lifestyle, spiritual, mindfulness, and community focus. Unfortunately, with the decimation of Tibetan Buddhism, there isn't a lot known about Tibetan yoga, and what is known has been adapted and created to fit modern yoga. It can be a hard class to find but you may be able to find classes titled as Tibetan yoga, Kum Nye, or OM yoga which are all adaptation of the original Tibetan yoga.

Each of these styles of yoga can help you achieve something in your life. Choose a couple to try. You might want to do a combination of classes, like one physical class and one spiritual one. Whichever way you choose, try to stick with just a couple of different styles, or focus on only one. Focusing on your particular practice gives you the opportunity to continue to grow in that one style. You'll gain a deeper awareness with each class, and you may find it easier to connect the physical with the spiritual if you stick to one pattern.

Chapter 9

Religious Yoga

In the past, yoga was considered to be a very spiritual practice. It was focused on the connection between the self and the universal self. Throughout this book, we've talked about the universal self, but what does that mean? To ancient yogis, the universal self was basically the part of us that is connected to all other living things on the planet. It was about the belief that we are all, in some way, connected to one another. It was later developed into the universal self as a way of differentiating our interconnectedness, and our individuality. This belief was almost entirely spiritual in nature.

This is distinctly different from a religion. A religion has rights and practices that are often focused on a deity. While some yoga traditions did connect with the local religious beliefs, yoga itself was distinct. It was adapted to fit the ideologies of the people who used it, and whether they used it for religious purposes or not, didn't change the basis of yoga as a form of spirituality, not a religion.

During the previous centuries, yoga wasn't linked with one religion per se. In fact, it predated most of the religions that were created from the *Vedas*. Instead, yoga was an aspect in many of the religions of the area. Buddhism, Jainism, and Hinduism all had yogic traditions that they followed and used. These traditions often overlapped with the religion. So the universal self became a specific deity, or not. There were also yoga practitioners who were not religious at all. So yoga was more of an additional aspect of spirituality that was added, or not, to religious beliefs of the time.

Today, yoga isn't considered to be religious. While yoga no longer has aspects of spirituality in most of the mainstream yoga classes, there are still some styles of yoga used today that are focused on spirituality. However, to practice yoga, you don't have to be a member of a particular faith. You don't even have to have a faith at all to practice yoga. Yoga practitioners aren't forced to worship a god or to pray to a particular deity. Because of this, and just like in the past, yoga can be used by people of all different faiths and beliefs. And, if you choose to, you can learn from the spiritual aspects of yoga that were part of the practice millenia ago. In this chapter, we will discuss the relation between yoga and beliefs, specifically religious or spiritual beliefs.

Yoga as a Spirituality

Yoga has always been considered a spirituality that focuses less on a deity and more on self-knowledge and wisdom. We can see aspects of that spirituality today in modern yoga practice. The meditative aspects of yoga, the control of the breath, even some movements can help a yoga practitioner grow to know themselves better. They can also use those skills to know their world better.

There are aspects of older yoga that call for specific actions or inactions. For instance, the Yoga Sutra talked about specific lifestyle actions, and while some of these were related to Hinduism, the actions often went beyond Hinduism into forming the world into a better place. The yamas and niyamas of ancient yoga discuss ethical actions of the day. These are actions that could still be used today to promote better wellbeing. While we did discuss this in brief before, let's recap a bit.

Yamas were things that you should not do. We shouldn't harm living creatures. We shouldn't lie or be untruthful. We shouldn't steal from others or envy what others have. We shouldn't be unfaithful in our relationships, and we shouldn't be attached to material things.

Niyamas were things that you should do. We should be pure of thought and clean in our body and lifestyle. We should be content with what we have and accept our world as it. We should persevere in our beliefs and actions. We should be self-reflective and aware of our actions. The last Niyama is religious in nature, speaking of contemplating a Supreme being. However, even if you remove that last niyama, the advice of the others is wise, and can be applied to our daily life.

This is just a small aspect of understanding the spirituality and lifestyle behind the yoga of the classical era. Following these actions could make the world a kinder place, and these are mostly about spirituality and less about religion.

The meditative aspects of yoga are also not religious in nature, and are instead about achieving personal growth and awareness. The pranayama and other meditative techniques associated with yoga, both past and present, were there with a goal of clearing the mind and quieting our anxieties and fears. Anyone who has regularly practiced mindfulness or meditation can point to how it helps us step away from our distracting thoughts. This doesn't mean that it's religious, more that it is a spiritual step that helps us be more aware of our present moment. Meditation and pranayama are used in many religions today as a way of connecting with a deity. But with yoga, it's often a way of just connecting with ourselves or connecting with that belief that we're all interconnected. So yoga is more closely related to a spirituality than a religion.

However, because of yoga's past connection with religions like Hinduism and Buddhism, many modern practitioners worry that yoga is a religion that will convert people away from other beliefs. So there have been concerns about promoting yoga in schools and public spaces, especially in the U.S., where Christianity is a religion with a lot of political influence. So let's break down some of the concerns that people have about yoga and how it can relate to different religions.

Christianity and Yoga

Christianity is a religion that is monotheistic. That is, Christians believe in one god but that one god has three faces, Jesus, God, and the Holy Spirit. Christianity is an Abrahamic religion, and developed in the Middle East with the descendants of Abraham before spreading with the Roman legions around Europe and Asia. There are many different groups of Christians, some more conservative than others. The beliefs of some Christians have clashed with yoga during the last 50 years, especially as yoga has become more popular.

In the U.S., many Christians grew concerned about the growth of yoga. After all, to those who don't know a lot about yoga, all we see is the connection to India and the religions of those areas. If you see a Swami or a monk practicing yoga, your first thought is that yoga is indeed religious. Many of the beliefs surrounding yoga are focused on this belief that yoga is a part of another religion. This can lead to misbeliefs about each part of yoga, from the asanas to the pranayamas.

However, if you study modern yoga, you'll find that yoga itself isn't inherently religious, but it can be closely tied to different religious practices. Yoga can even be tied with Christianity, if you choose to practice that way because yoga is highly adaptable. A Christian's practice can go in their own direction. There are some people who even practice yoga as a way to be nearer to God.

Brook Boon, a Christian yoga teacher and the founder of Holy Yoga puts it like this:

> I believe that we were created in the image of God, for the glory of God, for the worship of God. And all of the things that we're talking about in terms of Western yoga that we practice in gyms and in studios -pranayama, meditation, and asanas- all three of those things are addressed in the Bible. I believe that yoga is a spiritual discipline that draws you closer to God. And so, if that is true, then the intention of my heart trumps the posture of my body (Ferretti, 2017).

What Boon is suggesting, is that our intentions around yoga are what will define it for us. She even suggests that there are aspects of yoga that were mentioned in the Bible. Even if you look beyond the Bible, you can find that aspects of Christianity are very similar to the yamas of Raja yoga. For instance, Christianity also encourages nonviolence to all living beings, truthfulness, non-stealing, fidelity, and non-attachment to material things. Christianity can even connect with the niyamas, as these are rules contained in the Christian faith. So the way you use yoga could determine how you connect it to your faith.

That being said, if a Christian starts trying to follow the very spiritual aspects of yoga, especially Raja yoga, then they will come across some differences in yoga philosophy and Christianity. For example, Raja yoga and ones like it promote the idea of Karma. While karma in yoga is often considered the consequences of all actions, it can also be considered a part of the cycle of rebirth in some yoga traditions. This can go against Christian beliefs of one lifetime on Earth.

Other beliefs, like the fact that yoga is about self-realization can be considered as the opposite of Christianity's focus on God. However, some yogis, like Krishnamacharya, believed that self-realization was the same as God realization. So it really depends on the individual's perspective regarding self-realization and it's relation to their faith. All of this depends on their intentions behind practicing yoga.

There are those who use the meditative aspects of yoga to further their own faith in God. The two aren't incompatible. However, all of this depends on one's perspective. If you come from a fundamentalist Christian background, then it's likely that you'll be steered away from anything yoga related by the leaders of your faith. If you come from another Christian background, then you may find that many Christians like yourself encourage the use of yoga and meditation to help further your faith. So it really depends on your context, your faith, and the intention behind your practice.

If you're a Christian who plans on following the philosophy behind Raja yoga, then do so with the knowledge that it might challenge some parts of Christian doctrine. At the same time, it might enhance parts of your faith and personal relation-ship with God. Someone who is a Christian could practice yoga without compromising their faith in God. It all just depends on their intentions behind it. To sum up, yoga and Christianity aren't incompatible but it really depends on how you incorporate yoga into your faith (or if you leave it out of your faith entirely). If you're interested in learning more about Brooke Boon's work, check out her website and the yoga classes called Holy Yoga.

Islam and Yoga

Islam is a religion that is also monotheistic and, like Christianity, is an Abrahamic religion. In Islam, there is only one god, Allah, whose prophet Mohammed helped spread Islam across the Middle East. Islam was developed through the descendants of Abraham and grew in the Middle East before spreading across Asia and Southeast Asia. There are two groups of Muslims, Sunni and Shia. In some regions, Islam is more conservative than in others. The beliefs of some Muslims have clashed with yoga for a very long time.

As Islam spread to India in the Post-Classical Era, it's natural that yoga was one of the things that came up. Yoga and Islam eventually spread to all of Southeast Asia, and thus many people who practice Islam, also practice yoga in countries like Indonesia, Singapore and Malaysia. Yoga has also spread to Islamic countries in the Middle East, and is practiced by many Muslims. That being said, there are also some people against it.

In some Islamic countries, the practice of yoga is a crime, especially if it's used for spiritual reasons. This is because some people believe that yoga can turn people's eyes away from Allah and religious practices. Once again, just like in Christian arguments, yoga is often considered to be a purely Hindu religious practice. It's a difficult argument to win because it's so embedded with faith and belief.

There are many yogis who are Muslim and they connect yoga to their faith. Many people, even Imams (priests in Islam), have found that yoga can be very compatible if adapted to a Muslim audience. This is just like in the above discussion on Christianity. You can adapt parts of yoga to fit your beliefs. So Islam and yoga don't have to be incompatible.

From a philosophical point of view, there are many aspects of yoga that are similar to Muslim beliefs (yamas and niyamas). In fact you can go through the yamas and niyamas of yoga and find almost exactly the same guidelines in Islam. So you can find similarities like that. But many people also encourage leaving the spirituality out of yoga if you are practicing it as a Muslim. This means not doing the chants, and changing the clothing for women participants.

There are many Muslim yogis who incorporate yoga during Ramadan, the month long fast. This is because the fast calls Muslims to reflect on themselves and their relationship with Allah anyways, so adding a meditative aspect can help with that process. There are also some Muslims who see the daily prayer poses as very similar to yoga poses, offering the same benefits.

However, these explanations of how yoga and Islam connect will always depend on an individuals style of Islam. Conservative Muslims will not encourage the use of yoga, just as fundamentalist Christians don't.

Buddhism and Yoga

Buddhism is a religion that is non-religious. It's classified as a religion but religions are, by definition, focused on a deity or god. Buddhism is not a deity based religion, so it is both a religion and not one. Buddhism and yoga can connect together well, though there can be some issues with the very physicality of yoga and the focus on the self during yoga practices.

Because Buddhism and yoga began development during the same era and in some of the same areas, there are many overlapping beliefs, for example the eight limbs of Patanjali's Yoga Sutras are similar to the eightfold path of Buddhism. Yoga and Buddhism both encourage meditation, pranayama, closing the senses, etc. So many aspects of yoga can be similar to Buddhism. There are many Buddhists who practice yoga to the benefit of their faith.

Starting with the postures of yoga, many Buddhists find that the movements of asana can help before meditation or as a way to ease into meditation. There is an opportunity to use the asanas as a meditative tool, like it was originally intended centuries ago. Many Buddhists use the sitting postures of yoga to help them find settlement when sitting during meditation. The pranayamas of yoga can also help with increasing the comfort level and bring awareness inside instead of outside. So there is a little more connection between the spirituality of yoga and Buddhism then there is between some other religions.

There can be some conflicts between practicing yoga and Buddhism. Buddhism does emphasis the non-self or non-attachment to the self. The physicality of modern yoga can present the opposite problem as it is very body and self focused. However, that doesn't mean that Buddhism is incompatible with yoga. Instead, many practitioners can turn the focus away from those aspects of yoga and look at the ways it furthers their own faiths and beliefs.

In other countries, many Buddhist schools have developed their own takes on yoga and its use in Buddhism. Zen Buddhism and Tibetan Buddhism tend to have their own yoga activities.

Phillip Moffitt, a Buddhist and a member of the Spirit Rock Teachers Council, had this to say about Buddhism and yoga:

> I also think it is important to note that neither of these traditions is conversion-oriented. When I am teaching buddhad-harma, I do so without any agenda that people should become something different. It is truly the Buddha's indication to see for yourself, and that same quality is there in the people who are teaching the Patanjali [Yoga] Sutras. Both traditions offer a space for people to have their own experience, whether they are a Christian or a Jew or whatever. It is an exploration of the mind-body. (Where Buddhism & Yoga Meet, 2016).

This explanation connects to basically everything I explained before. Yoga isn't trying to convert people to a belief system. Instead, you can take from it what you want and use it to meet your own needs.

Following Your Own Path

As mentioned before, yoga is highly adaptable. This means that it can mean what it means to you. You don't have to follow what your yoga teacher is telling you and you can choose to follow your own yoga path. Each class can be adapted to you and what you are looking for from yoga. If you are looking for the spiritual aspects of yoga, then know that ahead of time and approach each yoga class from that perspective. There are teachers who will use phrases or have images that are connected to Hinduism or Buddhism in class, but that doesn't mean that you have to follow what your teacher does in regards to that if you are nonreligious. Your yoga practice is your own. If there is an aspect of your class that isn't for you, then don't participate with that part. For example, if you're a Christian and don't want to do the chants, then don't do them and come to class knowing ahead of time what you want to get out of the yoga class. If you are Buddhist but there are a lot of deity-related parts of the class, then you don't have to participate in those parts that don't agree with you. No one is going to force you to follow the doctrine of the teacher or their religious beliefs. Yoga will always be a safe space for people of all faiths and backgrounds. So choose your path in yoga and set your intention before stepping into class, especially if you want to connect yoga to your faith or religion.

The intentionality behind yoga can be connected to other faiths or non-beliefs. It doesn't matter whether you are religious or not, yoga can work for you. You can be an Atheist who practices yoga purely for the meditations and asanas without any connection to spirituality. You could be someone who wants to be fully engaged in the spirituality of yoga. You could be someone who wants to focus on the benefits of yoga while practicing your own faith. Or you could be someone who wants to incorporate your faith, whatever it is, into your yoga practice. Yoga can fit you without changing your religion or faith. It all just depends on your intentions with practicing yoga.

Before ending this chapter, I want to discuss a little about Hinduism and yoga. I didn't give Hinduism a set area in this chapter because yoga was so closely tied to Hinduism in the past and is still practiced as part of Hinduism. What I want to discuss is the Hindu view of yoga in the West. There are many Hindu's who are upset that yoga in the West is mostly physical instead of spiritual. They believe that people are missing out on some of the key benefits of yoga. This isn't a push to convert people to Hinduism but rather encouragement for people to see the spiritual aspects of yoga applied to their lives. Hopefully, this book can help you see the spiritual benefits of yoga, if you choose to pursue that path.

Conclusion

Yoga has made an amazing journey over the millenia. From an oral tradition that started in 5000 BCE to a modern practice today, yoga has had an impact on cultures around the world.

The ancient form of yoga was entirely spiritual in nature. It focused on the connection between man and the world around him. It was used to ask questions about life and to better understand God, the universe, and the self. Being a meditative and mindful practice, yoga was the way of joining together the human spirit and the universal spirit. As the religions of the time developed, so too did yoga and its understanding of the universal spirit. In Hinduism, the universal spirit became connected to Brahma while in other traditions, it was connected to different gods, goddess, or a non-deity.

Yoga started incorporating physical postures slowly, as a way to better prepare for meditation and to be comfortable during the meditation. Again, the focus was entirely on spirituality, with some more focus on philosophy and lifestyle coming into relevancy. From this meditative form of yoga, called Raja yoga, came multiple branches of yoga. The main ones were Bhakti yoga, Karma yoga, Jnana yoga, Hatha yoga, and Tantra yoga.

Bhakti yoga was considered the greatest yoga of all because it understood the value of loving kindness and relationships between practitioners and the universe or supreme being. It was the yoga of the heart.

Karma yoga was also highly regarded as it focused on improving the lives of others. It was a way of being ethical and, in a way, indifferent to the consequences of actions. This didn't mean that it promoted cruelty with disregard. Instead, it promoted ethical decision making and nonattachment to the consequences. The practitioner couldn't be biased when making decisions. They simply had to make the best decision offered to them. Karma yoga was the yoga of work.

Jnana yoga was the most difficult form of yoga, as it focused on gaining knowledge and wisdom of the self versus the universal self. It was a deeply meditative practice and was used constantly as a part of life. Jnana yoga was the yoga of the mind and knowledge.

Hatha yoga was a physical version of yoga. Each pose and position was used to achieve greater meditation and control the prana, the life force, within the body. Hatha yoga had practices that were difficult for many people outside of yoga to understand, and thus it wasn't treated well during the early eras. Hatha yoga was the yoga of the body.

Tantra yoga was distinct from the other forms of yoga as it didn't want to escape suffering. Instead, Tantra yogis believed that suffering was a part of life and thus needed to be experienced, not overcome. They also believed that the self and the universal self were one in the same, without separation. Tantra yoga was the yoga of ritual.

From these first forms of yoga came many others. As the centuries passed, yoga became more focused on physicality instead of spirituality. By the middle of the 20th century, yoga was almost entirely physical in practice. The movements and positions took precedence over meditation and mindfulness. Today, many people know yoga only as a physical exercise and sport, though the mindful and spiritual aspects of its roots haven't been forgotten.

I highly recommend you explore the variations of yoga out there. There are so many to choose from and you can learn about many of the different parts of yoga from them. If you choose to develop your spirituality and physical body through yoga, prepare yourself for personal growth. There is a lot to learn from such a rich history.

To bring this book to a close, I recommend that you continue your studies on yoga by reading some of these books:

- The Bhagavad-Gita. There are many translations of this book available for purchase, but you'll also probably find a copy at your local library. If you remember from earlier in this book, the Bhagavad Gita is a story within the *Mahabharata*. The story is about Krishna teaching a young prince about yoga. It's honestly very beautifully written. A good translated option is the one written by Eknath Easwaran. It's fairly easy to read and it includes notes about the translation and some meaning behind the stories. Another good option is the translation by Stephen Mitchell. This version is very enjoyable to read and is easy to follow along with. Whichever translation you choose, make sure that you give the Bhagavad-Gita a good read. And then read it again. I swear, every time I read it I learn something new.

- *Autobiography of a Yogi*. This book was

written by Paramahansa Yogananda, one of the yogis who spread yoga to America. It's considered one of the best spiritual classics in the world, and is very inspiring. If you want to learn more about the rich history of yoga and meditation, as well as the path Yogananda took, then I highly recommend that you read this book. It has inspired many people but beyond that, it can provide you with a new aspect of your own yoga practice. You can easily find a copy to purchase at your local bookstore, or online. You may even be able to find a copy at your local library.

- The Yoga Sutras. These were written by Patanjali but you'll have to purchase the translation unless you know Sanskrit. The Yoga Sutras are a collection of short poems based on yoga. They're no more than a few words long, but can have a really deep meaning. My favorite translation is the one by I.K. Taimni titled *The Science of Yoga*. This translation has a great interpretation of the Yoga Sutras and very good commentary too. It's easy to read and follow, though you'll have to take the time to interpret the

Sutras for yourself, since everyone walks away with a little difference in their understanding of them. This is a book you'll want to read again and again, as your understanding of the Sutras will change as time passes.

- *Light on Iyengar.* This book was written by B.K.S. Iyengar, the founder of Iyengar yoga. If you want to read a book that will teach you the reasons behind yoga and encourage you to practice, then this is the book for you. There is a lot of sound advice here but also some really good philosophical leanings about the nature of man and the importance of loving kindness. You can find a copy of this book from any online book retailer.

And there you have it. The history of yoga. I hope you've enjoyed reading this book. I also hope it has inspired you to consider the multiple aspects of yoga and consider practicing it yourself in the future. We'll end this book like any yoga class ends, with a kind and gentle, "Namaste."

References

Adler, M. (2012, April 11). To Some Hindus, Modern Yoga Has Lost Its Way. Retrieved from https://www.npr.org/2012/04/11/150352063/to-some-hindus-modern-yoga-has-lost-its-way.

Banhatti, G. S. (2015). Life and philosophy of Swami Vivekananda. New Delhi: Atlantic Publishers & Distributors (P) Ltd.

Bhutkar, M. V., Bhutkar, P. M., Taware, G. B., & Surdi, A. D. (2011). How Effective Is Sun Salutation in Improving Muscle Strength, General Body Endurance and Body Composition? Asian Journal of Sports Medicine, 2(4). doi: 10.5812/asjsm.34742

Burgin, T., Ava, Mueller, A., Catherine, Doran, A., Padget, B., ... Egon. (2014, November 20). Jnana Yoga: The Yoga of Wisdom. Retrieved from https://www.yogabasics.com/learn/jnana-yoga-the-yoga-of-wisdom/.

Carrico, M. (2007, August 28). The Branches of the Yoga Tree. Retrieved from https://www.yogajournal.com/practice/the-branches-of-yoga.

Carrico, M. (2007, August 28). Get to Know the Eight Limbs of Yoga. Retrieved from https://www.yogajournal.com/practice/the-eight-limbs.

Chapple, C. K. (2006). Yoga and the Mahabharata: Engaged Renouncers. Journal of Vaishnava Studies, 14(2), 103–114.

Cook, J. (2007, August 28). Find Your Match Among the Many Types of Yoga. Retrieved from https://www.yogajournal.com/practice/not-all-yoga-is-created-equal.

Daly, L. A., Haden, S. C., Hagins, M., Papouchis, N., & Ramirez, P. M. (2015). Yoga and Emotion Regulation in High School Students: A Randomized Controlled Trial. Evidence-Based Complementary and Alternative Medicine, 2015, 1–8. doi: 10.1155/2015/794928

Farinatti, P. T., Rubini, E. C., Silva, E. B., & Vanfraechem, J. H. (2014). Flexibility of the elderly after one-year practice of yoga and calisthenics. International Journal of Yoga Therapy, 24, 71–77. Retrieved from https://www.ncbi.nlm.nih.gov/pubmed/25858653

Ferretti, A. (2012, March 1). Yoga As a Religion? Retrieved from https://www.yogajournal.com/yoga-101/beyond-belief.

Frawley, D. (n.d.). Pratyahara: Yoga's forgotten limb. Retrieved from https://yogainternational.com/article/view/pratyahara-yogas-forgotten-limb.

Ghose, A., & Pershad. (1990). An introduction to the Vedas and the Upanishads: a compilation from the writings of Sri Aurobindo. Hyderabad, India: Sri Aurobindo Society, Hyderabad Branch.

Harvard Health Publishing. (n.d.). Yoga – Benefits Beyond the Mat. Retrieved from https://www.health.harvard.edu/staying-healthy/yoga-benefits-beyond-the-mat.

Harvard Health Publishing. (n.d.). Yoga for anxiety and depression. Retrieved from https://www.health.harvard.edu/mind-and-mood/yoga-for-anxiety-and-depression.

Heileman, J. (n.d.). Why breath matters. Retrieved from https://yogainternational.com/article/view/why-breath-matters-and-how-to-breathe-well-in-yoga-class.

Holcombe, K. (2015, November 17). The Yoga Sutra: Your Guide To Living Every Moment. Retrieved from https://www.yogajournal.com/yoga-101/yoga-sutra-guide-to-living-every-moment.

Isaacs, N. (2007, August 28). Tantra Rising. Retrieved from https://www.yogajournal.com/yoga-101/tantra-rising.

Isaacs, N. (2008, July 16). What is Bhakti Yoga? Why You Should Try the Yoga of Devotion. Retrieved from https://www.yogajournal.com/yoga-101/bhakti-yoga-love-devotion-relationship.

Jivamukti Yoga Center New York: Yoga Classes & Vegan Café Near Union Square. (n.d.). Retrieved from https://jivamuktiyoga.com/.

Link, R. (2017). 13 Benefits of yoga that are supported by science. Retrieved from https://www.healthline.com/nutrition/13-benefits-of-yoga.

Lion's Roar Staff. (2019, July 24). Where Buddhism & Yoga Meet. Retrieved from https://www.lionsroar.com/buddhism-and-yoga-where-the-paths-cross/.

Mallinson, J., & Singleton, M. (2017). Roots of yoga. London: Penguin Books.

McCall, T., & M.d. (2007, August 28). 38 Health Benefits of Yoga. Retrieved from https://www.yogajournal.com/lifestyle/count-yoga-38-ways-yoga-keeps-fit.

Nir, S. M. (2012, April 8). Seeking to Clear a Path Between Yoga and Islam. Retrieved from https://www.nytimes.com/2012/04/09/nyregion/in-queens-seeking-to-clear-a-path-between-yoga-and-islam.html.

Overview. (2018, December 25). Retrieved from https://triyoga.com/triyoga/overview/.

Paul, G. (n.d.). The Ultimate Science of Yoga . Retrieved from http://www.cs.albany.edu/~goutam/ScYogaCamera.pdf.

Pizer, A. (2019, July 17). Get Fierce With This Warrior Pose Sequence for Yoga Home Practice. Retrieved from https://www.verywellfit.com/get-fierce-with-this-sequence-of-warrior-poses-3567198.

Pizer, A. (2019, July 31). Start Your Yoga Practice With a Sun Salutation Warm up Sequence. Retrieved from https://www.verywellfit.com/illustrated-stepbystep-sun-salutation-3567187.

Pose Finder. (2017, April 5). Retrieved from https://www.yogajournal.com/pose-finder.

Razza, R. A., Bergen-Cico, D., & Raymond, K. (2015). Enhancing Preschoolers' Self-Regulation Via Mindful Yoga. Journal of Child and Family

Studies, 24(2), 372–385. doi: 10.1007/s10826-013-9847-6

Rosen, R. (2012). Original Yoga. Random House USA.

Ruiz, F. P. (2007, August 28). Krishnamacharya's Legacy: Modern Yoga's Inventor. Retrieved from https://www.yogajournal.com/yoga-101/krishnamacharya-s-legacy.

Samaveda. (2019, November 22). Retrieved from https://en.wikipedia.org/wiki/Samaveda#Cultural_influence.

Singleton, M. (2010). Yoga body the origins of modern posture practice. Oxford: Oxford University Press.

Singleton, M. (2011, February 4). The Ancient & Modern Roots of Yoga. Retrieved from https://www.yogajournal.com/yoga-101/yoga-s-greater-truth.

The Good Body. (2019, October 28). Yoga Statistics: Staggering Growth Shows Ever-increasing Popularity. Retrieved from https://www.thegoodbody.com/yoga-statistics/.

Tigunait, P. R. (n.d.). Seeing yoga in context. Retrieved from https://yogainternational.com/ article/view/seeing-yoga-in-context.

Tigunait, P. R. (n.d.). Q&A: What is the Vedic tradition? . Retrieved from https:// yogainternational.com/article/view/qa-what-is-the-vedic-tradition.

Violatti, C. (2019, November 22). Upanishads. Retrieved from https://www.ancient.eu/ Upanishads/.

Violatti, C. (2019, November 21). The Vedas. Retrieved from https://www.ancient.eu/ The_Vedas/.

Woodyard, C. (2011). Exploring the therapeutic effects of yoga and its ability to increase quality of life. International Journal of Yoga, 4(2), 49. doi: 10.4103/0973-6131.85485

Yogananda, P. (2016). Autobiography Of A Yogi. S.l.: DIAMOND POCKET BOOKS.

Yogendra, H. J. (2019). Yoga for all: discovering the true essence of yoga. New Delhi: Rupa.